Children
with Spina Bifida

Children with Spina Bifida

Early Intervention and Preschool Programming

edited by

G. Gordon Williamson, Ph.D., OTR

Margery Szczepanski, M.A., OTR
Assistant Editor

with

Maryellen T. Aland, M.S., C.C.C./SP
Mary Caterson-Marshall, M.S., C.C.C./SP
Deirdre Cipriano, OTR
Marilyn Dunning, M.A.
Thomas W. Findley, Jr., M.D., Ph.D.
Flavia Bernardo Hall, M.A., C.C.C./SP
Kathryn Hessinger, LPT
Judy Kulick, R.N., B.S.N.
Samuel Laufer, M.D.
Lisa A. Leifer, LPT
Maureen Lukenda, A.C.S.W.
Grace A. Malone, OTR

Donna L. Picone, M.Ed., LPT
Marcia Reiff-Hacohen, OTR
Jeanne Rubin Kagan, M.A., OTR
Lisa N. Scher, LPT
Susan Shelby, LPT
Kathleen G. Storey, M.S., OTR
Thomas E. Strax, M.D.
Valorie R. Todd, M.A., OTR
Jeanne C. Winter, OTR
Shirley Zeitlin, Ed.D.
Lucia Zubizarreta, M.A., LPT

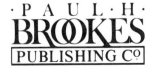

·P A U L·H·
BROOKES
PUBLISHING CO

Baltimore • London

Paul H. Brookes Publishing Co.
Post Office Box 10624
Baltimore, Maryland 21285-0624

Typeset by Brushwood Graphics Studio, Baltimore, Maryland.
Manufactured in the United States of America by
The Maple Press Company, York, Pennsylvania.

Drawings by Kathleen Gray Farthing.

Photographs by Stephen T. Krencicki (except for Figures 3.6, 3.12,
3.26–3.28, 5.1, 5.3, and 5.6).

Library of Congress Cataloging-in-Publication Data
Children with spina bifida.
  Bibliography: p.
  Includes index.
  1. Spina bifida—Psychological aspects.   2. Perceptual-motor learn-
ing.   3. Spina bifida—Patients—Care and treatment.   4. Spina
bifida—Patients—Transportation.   5. Spina bifida—Patients—Family
relationships.   6. Spina bifida—Patients—Education.   I. Williamson,
G. Gordon.   II. Szczepanski, Margery.   [DNLM: 1. Education,
Special.   2. Spina Bifida—rehabilitation.   WE 730 C536]
RJ496.S74C48   1987   362.1'97482   86-20748
ISBN 0-933716-71-0

Contents

Contributors

Nursing
Judy Kulick, R.N., B.S.N.
Pediatric Rehabilitation Department
Johnson Rehabilitation Institute
John F. Kennedy Medical Center
2050 Oak Tree Road
Edison, NJ 08820

Occupational Therapy
Deirdre Cipriano, OTR
Pediatric Rehabilitation Department
Johnson Rehabilitation Institute
John F. Kennedy Medical Center
2050 Oak Tree Road
Edison, NJ 08820

Grace A. Malone, OTR
Pediatric Rehabilitation Department
Johnson Rehabilitation Institute
John F. Kennedy Medical Center
2050 Oak Tree Road
Edison, NJ 08820

Marcia Reiff-Hacohen, OTR
Occupational Therapy Department
Blythedale Children's Hospital
Valhalla, NY 10595

Jeanne Rubin Kagan, M.A., OTR
Department of Rehabilitation Services
Newington Children's Hospital
181 East Cedar Street
Newington, CN 06111

Margery Szczepanski, M.A., OTR
Pediatric Rehabilitation Department
Johnson Rehabilitation Institute
John F. Kennedy Medical Center
2050 Oak Tree Road
Edison, NJ 08820

Valorie R. Todd, M.A., OTR
Pediatric Rehabilitation Department
Johnson Rehabilitation Institute
John F. Kennedy Medical Center
2050 Oak Tree Road
Edison, NJ 08820

Jeanne C. Winter, OTR
Pediatric Rehabilitation Department
Johnson Rehabilitation Institute
John F. Kennedy Medical Center
2050 Oak Tree Road
Edison, NJ 08820

Kathleen G. Storey, M.S., OTR
Pediatric Occupational Therapy
St. Barnabas Medical Center
Old Short Hills Road
Livingston, NJ 07039

G. Gordon Williamson, Ph.D., OTR
Pediatric Rehabilitation Department
Johnson Rehabilitation Institute
John F. Kennedy Medical Center
2050 Oak Tree Road
Edison, NJ 08820

Orthopaedic Surgery

Samuel Laufer, M.D.
Pediatric Orthopedic Associates, P.A.
585 Cranbury Road
East Brunswick, NJ 08816

Physical Therapy

Kathryn Hessinger, LPT
Pediatric Rehabilitation
Monmouth Medical Center
300 Second Avenue
Long Branch, NJ 07740

Lisa A. Leifer, LPT
Private Practice
350 Rahway Road
Edison, NJ 08820

Donna L. Picone, M.Ed., LPT
Pediatric Rehabilitation Department
Johnson Rehabilitation Institute
John F. Kennedy Medical Center
2050 Oak Tree Road
Edison, NJ 08820

Lisa N. Scher, LPT
Pediatric Rehabilitation Department
Johnson Rehabilitation Institute
John F. Kennedy Medical Center
2050 Oak Tree Road
Edison, NJ 08820

Susan Shelby, LPT
Private Practice
85 Lindsley Avenue
West Orange, NJ 07052

Lucia Zubizarreta, M.A., LPT
Pediatric Rehabilitation Department
Johnson Rehabilitation Institute
John F. Kennedy Medical Center
2050 Oak Tree Road
Edison, NJ 08820

Psychology

Shirley Zeitlin, Ed.D.
Pediatric Rehabilitation Department
Johnson Rehabilitation Institute
John F. Kennedy Medical Center
2050 Oak Tree Road
Edison, NJ 08820

Rehabilitation Medicine

Thomas W. Findley, Jr., M.D.,
Ph.D.
Pediatric Rehabilitation
Rhode Island Hospital
Providence, RI 02902

Thomas E. Strax, M.D.
Rehabilitation Medicine
Johnson Rehabilitation Institute
John F. Kennedy Medical Center
James Street
Edison, NJ 08818

Social Work

Maureen Lukenda, A.C.S.W.
Center for Infant Development
Elizabeth Board of Education
630 South Street
Elizabeth, NJ 07202

Special Education

Marilyn Dunning, M.A.
Pediatric Rehabilitation Department
Johnson Rehabilitation Institute
John F. Kennedy Medical Center
2050 Oak Tree Road
Edison, NJ 08820

Speech-Language Pathology

Maryellen T. Aland, M.S.,
C.C.C./SP
Pediatric Rehabilitation Department
Johnson Rehabilitation Institute
John F. Kennedy Medical Center
2050 Oak Tree Road
Edison, NJ 08820

Flavia Bernardo Hall, M.A.,
C.C.C./SP
Pediatric Rehabilitation Department
Johnson Rehabilitation Institute
John F. Kennedy Medical Center
2050 Oak Tree Road
Edison, NJ 08820

Mary Caterson-Marshall, M.S.,
C.C.C./SP
Pediatric Rehabilitation Department
Johnson Rehabilitation Institute
John F. Kennedy Medical Center
2050 Oak Tree Road
Edison, NJ 08820

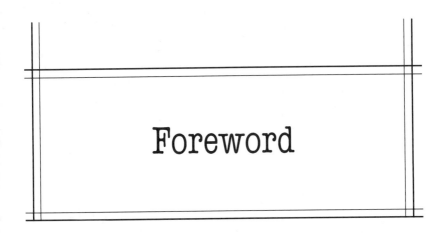

Foreword

SIGNIFICANT PROGRESS HAS OCCURRED IN THE LAST 20 YEARS IN THE MANAGEment of infants with myelomeningocele. Today's resources are enabling children with spina bifida to reach new levels of achievement in their development, learning, and quality of life. Medical advances have contributed to improved physical health, and expanded programs are providing early intervention and preschool services to these children and their families.

There has long been a need for a publication that offers in-depth assistance to the practitioner in the areas of assessment and intervention. This book meets such a need and is therefore truly unique. It takes an interdisciplinary approach that emphasizes services for the child *and* family.

Although *Children with Spina Bifida* by Dr. Williamson and his colleagues is targeted to a specific condition, the book has a wealth of information that is pertinent to children with other types of developmental disabilities. It is a contribution to the field that promises to have an important impact.

Howard A. Rusk, M.D.
Founder, Rusk Institute of Rehabilitation Medicine
Distinguished University Professor
New York University

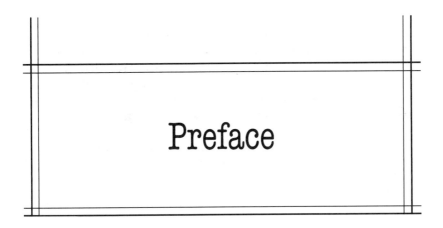

Preface

THE INTENT OF THIS BOOK IS TO PROVIDE A COMPREHENSIVE, PRACTICAL GUIDE for the delivery of early intervention and preschool services to young children with spina bifida and their families. Since these children vary greatly, this volume focuses primarily on the needs of children with myelomeningocele who have neuromotor and associated problems that require special medical, therapeutic, and educational intervention. The book is written for professionals who work in clinics, hospitals, school systems, child care centers, and rehabilitation agencies as well as students in training at colleges and universities. However, many parents may find the content helpful in understanding their child and the nature of his or her educational and therapeutic program. Such shared awareness by parents and professionals will hopefully facilitate a truly cooperative partnership.

The scope of the book is broad in its coverage but explicit in reporting the knowledge and skills required by the practitioner. Every effort is made to reflect exemplary professional practices based on the most current research in the field. Procedures for interdisciplinary assessment and intervention address the following areas: postural control and mobility, perceptual-motor skills, speech and language, activities of daily living, and unique educational requirements. Specific attention is directed to physical positioning, wheelchair use, orthopaedic management, bracing, and health-related considerations (e.g., skin care, bowel and bladder management, nutrition). Methods, materials, and intervention strategies are discussed for each content area.

Fundamental to the philosophy of this book is an appreciation of the uniqueness of each child. Therefore, the presented content must be selectively interpreted as to its relevance for a particular infant, toddler, or preschooler. A comprehensive interdisciplinary assessment, in close collaboration with the parents, is essential for designing a personalized service plan that enhances the developmental competence of the child and the coping resources of the family.

The authors of this book represent all of the major rehabilitative, educational, and psychosocial disciplines in order to ensure complete coverage of the subject. They volunteered their time to this project with all royalties being donated to the Spina Bifida Association of America. This book was written in part by the members of the Pediatric Rehabilitation Department of the Johnson Rehabilitation Institute, John F. Kennedy Medical Center, in Edison, New Jersey. The members of the department have had extensive experience in providing services to children with spina bifida and their families. Additional contributions to the book were made by a pediatric orthopaedic surgeon and a physiatrist, each of whom have special expertise in this area. G. Gordon Williamson and Margery Szczepanski integrated the material into a cohesive document to avoid fragmentation by different authors addressing separate chapters.

Acknowledgments

GRATEFUL ACKNOWLEDGMENT IS EXTENDED TO THE CONTRIBUTING AUTHORS who were so willing to share of their time and talent. Margery Szczepanski deserves singular recognition for her critical role in all stages of the book's development—planning, organization, writing, and revision. The Spina Bifida Association of America was most supportive of this endeavor and provided helpful assistance through Betty Pieper, former chairperson of its Publications Committee.

Kathleen Gray Farthing provided the illustrations, and Stephen T. Krencicki was responsible for the photography with assistance from the staff of the Pediatric Rehabilitation Department, Johnson Rehabilitation Institute, John F. Kennedy Medical Center. Gratitude is expressed to the children (especially Stephanie and Ryan) and their families for permission to use the photographs. Evelyn Katrak was instrumental in preparing the manuscript for publication, and Kathy Conway was tireless in typing its many drafts. Special thanks are also due to Melissa A. Behm of Brookes Publishing Company for her highly professional guidance. Sincere appreciation is extended to each and every one of these remarkable individuals.

To Patricia Gilchrist and Joseph Sherber
who take chances so that the
future will be better.

Children
with Spina Bifida

◇ CHAPTER 1 ◇

Children with Spina Bifida and their Families

SPINA BIFIDA IS A GENERAL TERM THAT ENCOMPASSES A WIDE VARIETY OF neural tube defects. It is used to describe children who have no neurological dysfunction as well as children with mild to very severe handicaps. This chapter provides an introduction to the nature of spina bifida and addresses issues related to the delivery of services to young children and their families.

THE NATURE OF SPINA BIFIDA

Spina bifida means cleft spine—a spine "split" because the bones of the spinal column (the vertebrae) fail to enclose the spinal cord during the first trimester of pregnancy. This condition is referred to as a neural tube defect (lesion). The malformation occurs between the third and sixth week of gestation, before many women have confirmed their pregnancy.

During the first month of normal gestation, the flat ribbon of tissue that runs down the middle of the embryo develops a deepening groove. Its edges grow up and around until they meet, forming a tube. This neural tube eventually differentiates into the brain and spinal cord. Supportive and protective tissues (meninges) develop to enclose the spinal cord and brain. Later, the bony vertebrae form to surround the spinal cord and the skull forms to protect the brain. In spina bifida, some section of the neural tube fails to fuse or close, resulting in abnormal development of the meninges, nerves, and vertebrae (Anderson & Spain, 1977).

There are three types of spina bifida (see Figure 1.1). The most common type, and the least severe, is *spina bifida occulta.* In this condition, there is an abnormal opening in the spine because the back arches of the vertebrae do not fuse. The spinal cord and nerves are typically not damaged, and neurological functioning is usually intact. At the site of the defect, there may be a dimple on the skin, tufts of hair, or nothing visible at all. Individuals with spina bifida occulta may not even be aware that they have the condition. In a minority of

1

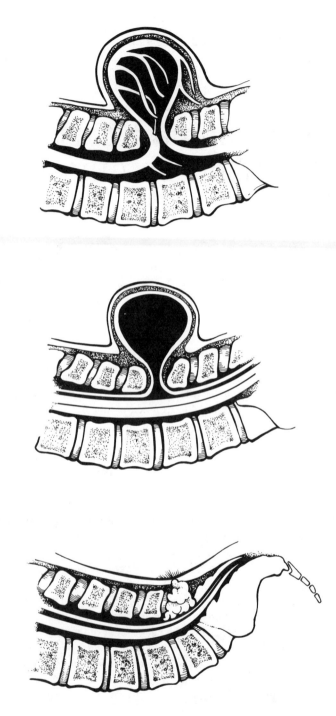

Figure 1.1. Three types of spina bifida. From left to right: spina bifida occulta, meningocele, and myelomeningocele.

cases, however, there can be problems in bowel or bladder continence and in motor control of the legs (Brocklehurst, 1976).

Meningocele is second in severity, and it is the least common of the three types. The meninges (protective coverings) are pushed out through the opening in the vertebrae and form a sac (herniation), which is usually covered by normal skin. This sac, called the meningocele, contains the meninges and cerebrospinal fluid. The fluid bathes and protects the nerve cells by circulating freely. In this type of spinal bifida, the spinal cord remains intact. Corrective surgery is performed to reposition the meninges and remove the sac. After surgery, the child often has no neurological deficit, although in some cases sensory and motor handicaps may be present.

Myelomeningocele (pronounced mý-el-lo-men-ing-go-seal) is the second most common and the most serious type of spina bifida; it usually causes a significant degree of impairment. The vertebrae fail to fuse and the meninges and the spinal cord protrude to form a sac. In such cases, the spinal cord fails to develop properly, and the spinal nerves are damaged. The neurological deficit is not confined to the specific site where the sac is exposed. The spinal cord below the level of the sac is usually abnormal, and the cord is frequently impaired for several spinal segments above the sac.

Meningocele and myelomeningocele are occasionally grouped together under the label spina bifida cystica. The term myelodysplasia is a general term that refers to defective formation of the spinal cord.

Level of Lesion

The spinal cord is divided into four major segments—cervical, thoracic, lumbar, and sacral—with 31 symmetrically arranged pairs of spinal nerves exiting from the spinal column to innervate (supply nerve stimulation to) the body. There are 8 cervical nerve pairs, in the neck; 12 thoracic nerve pairs, in the region of the rib cage; 5 lumbar nerve pairs, in the area of the low back; 5 sacral nerve pairs, near the base of the spine; and 1 coccygeal nerve pair, at the end of the cord. Therefore, 31 spinal nerves provide sensory and motor innervation to each side, left and right, of the body. (The motor and sensory levels of the spinal cord are presented in Appendix A.)

A lesion can occur at any point on the spinal cord, although it is most frequently found in the lumbosacral region (Hammock & Milhorat, 1982). The level of the lesion is medically determined by the site of the herniation on the cord and the resulting damage to the spinal nerves exiting from that area of the spine. Different levels of lesion result in specific patterns of motor paralysis and loss of sensation. For example, a myelomeningocele at the level of the twelfth thoracic vertebra or above results in a paralysis of the trunk and lower extremities. That is, muscle function in the trunk and legs is weak or absent. Children with such a lesion have total or partial loss of sensation for touch, pain, pressure, and temperature below the level of the lesion, as well as bowel and bladder incontinence. In contrast, spinal cord damage in the lower trunk (third or fourth lumbar vertebra) results in some muscle control in the upper part of the legs, but no motor activity in the lower area of the legs.

There is wide variation in the motor and sensory deficits of children with myelomeningocele. There may be asymmetry in innervation between the two sides of the body as well as a difference between the motor and sensory levels of innervation. The motor paralysis may present a clinical picture of both upper and lower motor neuron lesions (i.e., flaccidity and spasticity). It is important to remember that in addition to the spinal defect, there can be brain anomalies such as the Arnold-Chiari malformation in the brain stem.

Incidence and Etiology

The prevalence of neural tube defects has varied over time and by geographical location. Wolraich (1983) has reported that the incidence of spina bifida in the United States is .7–1 case per 1,000 live births. Various studies have suggested a trend toward a decreasing occurrence of the condition (Crowe et al., 1985; Windham & Edmonds, 1982). However, spina bifida (meningocele and my-elomeningocele) remains the second most common specific birth defect after trisomy 21, a type of Down syndrome (Myers, 1984). Myelomeningocele is four to five times more common than meningocele (Bleck, 1975).

The specific causes of spina bifida are not presently known. Research has suggested that genetic and environmental factors play an interactive role (Strassburg, Greenland, Portigal, & Sever, 1983). Indicators of a genetic component include a higher incidence of spina bifida in certain ethnic groups, which persists after migration, and the greater frequency of occurrence in certain family histories. Proposed environmental influences are innumerable (e.g., maternal fever in early pregnancy, viral infection, certain medications). There is some evidence that vitamin abnormality, particularly folic acid deficiency, may be related to spina bifida (Smithells et al., 1980); folate is involved in the synthesis of DNA, RNA, and certain amino acids. Although no single environmental agent has been identified, animal experiments indicate that a variety of toxic or mechanical agents acting on the fetus at the critical time may result in neural tube defects.

In summary, findings from research studies have not been uniform and the cause of spina bifida remains unknown. Most likely, it is some combination of interacting genetic and environmental factors.

Prenatal Screening

There are a number of procedures available for the prenatal detection of neural tube defects. One approach is to test the level of alpha-fetoprotein (AFP) in the expectant mother's blood. AFP is produced in the liver of all individuals, including the developing fetus, which normally has a high concentration of AFP in its blood serum. In the case of an open neural tube defect such as myelomeningocele, an excessive amount of AFP passes into the amniotic fluid and into the maternal bloodstream. A blood sample from the mother showing an abnormally high concentration of AFP (a "positive" result) may indicate the possibility of an open neural tube defect. Usually the blood test is conducted 15–22 weeks after the last menstrual period (Chappell, 1982). A positive result of AFP screening may also occur with the presence of twins or with faulty calculation of the duration of pregnancy. When an elevated level of AFP is detected, further investigation, such as diagnostic ultrasonography and amniocentesis, is required.

Amniocentesis involves inserting a needle into the amniotic sac and extracting a small quantity of amniotic fluid. To avoid touching the fetus or placenta with the needle and thus causing injury, the physician employs sonography (ultrasound) during this procedure. Sound waves are directed toward the fetus and are reflected back to an instrument that outlines the form of the fetus on a screen. The extracted amniotic fluid is analyzed to obtain a quantitative measurement of the level of AFP (Swinyard, 1980).

Other prenatal tests are also used to detect spina bifida. An amniogram can be performed, in which a contrast medium is injected into the amniotic sac and an X ray is taken. Another procedure employs a fiber optic microscope. A fine tube that transmits light is introduced into the amniotic sac and allows direct visualization of the fetus.

If tests confirm that the fetus has spina bifida, the parents have the option to terminate the pregnancy or to carry the fetus to term. In the latter case, arrangements are often made to deliver the infant at a regional medical center where specialized services such as neurosurgery, to repair the back, and neonatal intensive care are available. The infant is frequently delivered by cesarean section in order to protect the protruding sac from further neurological damage.

SERVICES TO THE CHILD AND FAMILY

Children with spina bifida benefit from receiving services as early as possible. As a general rule, early intervention programs serve children under 36 months of age, and preschool programs serve children 3 and 4 years of age. These service models vary in their structure, format, and staffing. Effective programs at all ages require the participation of an interdisciplinary team working in close collaboration with the child and family. These programs share the following primary goals:

1. To promote the child's skills in all developmental areas—movement, cognition, communication, social-emotional and physical health, and adaptive behavior

2. To assist family members in adjusting to the impact of having a disabled child and in developing nurturing and caregiving skills
3. To increase the ability of the child and family to cope with the challenges and stresses of daily living

These goals are directed to both the child and the family. The presence of a handicapped child in the family creates additional stress that each family member must learn to manage (Gallagher, Bechman, & Cross, 1983; Kazak & Marvin, 1984). Families and individual members differ in their coping styles, available resources, and effectiveness in meeting the demands of daily living. It is important that professional services are family-oriented since the way in which the family copes influences the child's life outcome (Lavelle & Keogh, 1980), the family's overall functioning (Olsen & McCubbin, 1983; Seligman, 1985), and the parents' feelings of satisfaction and competence as caregivers (Turnbull, Summers, & Brotherson, 1983).

The child with spina bifida is viewed as an active participant in an ongoing learning process. An orientation that recognizes and values a child's unique personality, strengths, and needs is vital. With this orientation, developmental skills are fostered through opportunities for spontaneous exploration, peer interaction, experiential learning, and individualized therapeutic and educational programming. The child is also helped to learn adaptive strategies for managing his or her world. These experiences have optimal benefit when they are provided in as normal a social environment as possible.

It is disturbingly easy for professionals and parents to focus on the handicap and look for pathology by emphasizing what the child is not doing—not walking, not paying attention, not achieving developmental milestones. This perspective undermines a child's sense of self-worth and encourages an identity of being handicapped. In order to fulfill the handicapped role, the child may learn to behave like a "good patient": dependent on the expertise of the adult and always willing to adhere to the prescribed recommendations.

Over time, this orientation can lead to a state of learned helplessness (Greer & Wethered, 1984). Since the child is repeatedly being exposed to situations that are directed by others and beyond his or her control, the expectation eventually develops that his or her actions do not have a significant impact on environmental outcomes. This viewpoint may lead to passivity, dependency, and feelings of impotence. It also interferes with future learning, since the child is less likely to initiate actions to explore and solve problems.

Germain (1973) proposed a "life model" frame of reference as an alternative to a deficit-based model. This approach focuses on enhancing growth rather than correcting deficiencies. The developmental process is viewed as the acquisition of competencies through interaction with the physical, social, and cultural environment. The achievement of specific skills is related to psychological growth in the areas of self-esteem, impulse control, autonomous behavior, and interpersonal relations.

The life model is strongly influenced by Erikson's theory of the development of the ego through interactional tasks (1963). For example, he considers play an attempt by the child to synchronize bodily and social processes with a developing sense of self. Play reflects "the ego's need to master the various areas of life, and especially those in which the individual finds his self, his body and his social role wanting and trailing" (p. 211). Failure to play may contribute to continuing dependency, an inability to redirect fantasies and achieve individuation, excessive daydreaming, and poor emotional relations to others. Children with physical disabilities may be particularly vulnerable to this situation. It is essential, therefore, that sufficient opportunities be provided for the child to explore the rich dimensions of play and the interactions that play generates.

Another issue to consider is the many systems that have an impact on the child and family, including medical, therapeutic, educational, and social service systems. Typically, an array of professionals and agencies are involved. It is important that these systems coordinate their efforts to ensure a comprehensive and integrated approach. Collaboration is necessary to provide the conditions and resources that are conducive to the optimal functioning of the child and family. This responsibility necessitates a respect for the authoritative role of parents in decision making. Parents and professionals need to work cooperatively in planning and implementing any course of action.

Coping with Stress

How family members cope with daily demands and stressors is critical. Coping is defined as an active, adaptive process of using strategies to deal with one's world (Murphy & Moriarty, 1976). It is learned behavior that is influenced by one's development, temperament, prior experience, general level of competence, areas of vulnerability, and the demands of the environment. Experientially over time, one develops a unique coping style that reflects the habitual way in which one meets the opportunities and challenges of daily living (Zeitlin, 1985). That style includes the strategies one uses to meet personal needs and to adapt to the requirements of one's surroundings.

Coping behavior can be graded along a continuum of effectiveness, and it varies even within the individual depending on the situation. Adaptive coping behavior promotes solutions that assist in caring for oneself and/or responding appropriately to environmental demands. It fosters learning that can be generalized to other circumstances. In contrast, maladaptive coping behavior does not lead to satisfactory solutions. Although it may relieve immediate tension, it impedes new learning and eventually increases one's vulnerability to stress in the future.

It is important to understand the special needs of the family with a disabled child in order to facilitate their competencies and adaptive coping. Although all families are confronted with a series of developmental tasks, these families have more numerous and complex challenges (Murphy, 1982). They can be viewed as ordinary families under extraordinary stress. Not only must they cope with the demands of daily living, but they have to manage difficult periods that can readily assume crisis proportions if appropriate resources and support are not available. Peterson and Lippa (1978) have identified three major periods of stress that are commonly faced.

The first major period concerns issues related to diagnosis and the need for information. Expectant parents have an idealized image of the anticipated baby (Klaus & Kennell, 1976). During the early months after the birth, they must gradually adjust to the discrepancy between the idealized child and the actual infant, with all of its endearing and not so endearing characteristics. With the birth of an infant with myelomeningocele, the parents experience a period of mourning, in which they grieve the loss of the expected perfect child. This natural response places stress on their capacity to establish an emotional attachment to their infant.

At the same time, the family is struggling to understand the meaning and implications of their child's medical diagnosis. Prior to the birth of the child, many parents are totally unfamiliar with spina bifida. Despite the lack of previous information, they are immediately confronted with the need to make decisions regarding medical treatment and follow-up care. In some cases, the parents' decision to have the child treated and cared for at home is made regardless of the negative attitudes and pessimistic prognosis of professionals and family members. Endless questions arise to which the parents seek answers from the numerous health care personnel required by the child. These issues are related to the cause and severity of the disability as well as implications for the family (e.g., whether to consider having additional children; the impact of the disability on the child's siblings).

Socially, the parents may feel alienated by the response of family and friends to the birth of a child with a disability. Grandparents may be unable to offer support and assistance, as they too are experiencing a sense of loss and sorrow. Parents must then assist the grandparents in dealing with their reactions, in addition to working through their own feelings regarding the disability. The family may also be isolated from friends who feel inadequate in relating to them. The traditional welcoming rituals associated with the birth of a child (such as cards, flowers, visits, calls, parties, and pictures) may be limited or nonexistent. Thus, families may experience alienation at a time when their overwhelming need is for support.

During this time, families are also burdened with financial pressures resulting from the costs of the child's medical care. These costs include the expenses for the initial surgery and hospitalization (see Chapter 4) as well as follow-up medical and therapeutic intervention. Such costs may result in a long-term debt for families, many of whom must seek outside financial resources either from other family members or from larger social institutions.

The second major period of adjustment described by Peterson and Lippa (1978) covers the preschool through early teenage years, when issues related to socialization and school attendance come to the fore. During this period, parental concerns tend to focus on the child's social and cognitive development. Typically, a child's initial entry into the school system is a stressful event in the life of any family. For the parents of a child with myelomeningocele, adjustment to school entry may be complicated by their increased apprehension and residual feelings about the disability.

This period also places new demands on the family's problem-solving skills. Some parents may find themselves involved with an educational system that is largely unfamiliar with the special needs of the child with spina bifida. As a result, professionals providing services may appear to be uncomfortable with the child. This difficulty may be perceived by parents as institutional indifference, which forces them to assume an active role as advocates for their child's interests. Many parents lack adequate preparation for such a role, since appropriate educational services are taken for granted by the majority of the population.

Another area of stress encountered by some parents is the labeling of their child as learning disabled. Up to this point, the family may have focused on the physical disability; now they must shift attention to less visible problems. The formulation of an individualized education program (IEP) may be a painful process that once more revives personal issues related to the child's handicap and the parents' response to it.

During this period, parents are particularly concerned with the child's psychosocial development. By this age, the child is increasingly aware of his or her differences in comparison with peers. Questions arise regarding the disability that the parent must address with the child. This time is often extremely difficult, particularly if the parents' own feelings remain unresolved. Of course, the manner in which the family views the disability is critical in determining the child's attitude toward it.

The child's growing awareness is spurred by experiences outside the home involving interaction with other children. Although it may not be possible for the child with myelomeningocele to join fully in all the activities of peers, it is important that the child participate to the maximum extent of his or her capability. Nondisabled children may need subtle encouragement to include the physically handicapped child in activities, although inclusion is usually spontaneously initiated in young children. Persistent isolation from peers can lead to feelings of alienation and rejection, which, in turn, lead to the child's continued dependence on the family for socialization.

The third major period extends from adolescence through early adulthood. During this time, parents are concerned with their child's ability to function in society. Possibilities for future employment are explored, as well as the child's potential for independent living. As in earlier stages, the parents are forced to take a more active role—compared to parents of nonhandicapped children—in exploring appropriate resources to meet their offspring's changing needs. The level of emotional maturity and social integration of the young adult with spina bifida is largely dependent on the degree to which previous levels of development have been successfully achieved.

In summary, each period presents the parents with new challenges, which are sometimes experienced as times of crisis, followed by readjustment and stability. Parents do not reach a static stage of "acceptance"; rather, feelings change in relation to their ability to cope with the current situation. Many families need support during difficult periods to assist them in their coping efforts.

The Provision of Family-Oriented Services

A commitment to serving the needs of families can occur only in an atmosphere of mutual respect and open communication. The unnecessary use of technical language and jargon can lead to feelings of intimidation and misunderstanding. Parents are helped when they are confident that their viewpoint is valued. Initially, they may be hesitant to speak freely because of a fear of appearing uninformed or inadequate. It is particularly difficult for some parents to disagree openly with professionals. Although parents may privately question the assessment findings, educational classification, or program placement, they are not always able to bring their doubts to the attention of professionals.

Effective collaboration implies a partnership involving mutual give and take. Professionals need to beware of placing coercive pressures on families to conform to the set policies and procedures of the service organization. In addition, it is easy for professionals to view differences in personal values as challenges to their authority. Consequently, the professional may overuse psychological interpretations to explain the conflict in opinion or may consider such differences to be a reflection of parental maladjustment (Gliedman & Roth, 1980; Lipsky, 1985).

The importance of a relationship based on respect and trust cannot be overestimated. Without it, parents may actively or passively sabotage plans that they feel are inappropriate for their child. Ongoing communication of feelings, opinions, and priorities is essential for the collaborative development of a program that addresses the child's best interests. This section of the chapter highlights services that encourage family involvement.

The Intake Process The initial contact with an agency or school is critical in determining the nature of future interactions. It can be anticipated that this contact will produce significant anxiety in the family. It is important that the parents establish a relationship early with a social worker or other professional who can serve as a case manager throughout the intake and assessment process. Information should be shared regarding the available services, the sequential steps involved in determining the IEP or individualized service plan, the professionals to be involved, the parents' financial responsibilities (if applicable), and the role and rights of the parents during this process. An unhurried and thorough orientation to the program can greatly relieve the stress experienced by the parents and the child. It enables the family to perceive the service providers as receptive, rather than indifferent, to their needs; and it forms the basis for a positive relationship.

Case Coordination Parents may feel overpowered at having to deal with a multitude of professionals and trying to coordinate their services. A case manager can assist the development of an integrated and comprehensive plan of service that avoids duplication and fragmentation. Case coordination includes maintaining contact with other agencies serving the child and family. Through this interagency dialogue, gaps in needed resources can be identified and addressed. This is especially important during periods of transition, when a child is progressing from one program to another (e.g., discharged from an early intervention program to enter a preschool setting). This coordinating function is an ongoing process that is not limited to times of crisis.

Supportive Services Families can receive support through individual and group activities. Group activities are effective for providing information and emotional support to targeted family members—parents, siblings, and grandparents. Regularly scheduled parent discussion groups are based on a mutual aid model. Parents exchange experiences and work together to improve their capacity to cope with shared and individual problems. The mutual aid model emphasizes the ability of group members to offer helpful support to one another. A social worker, psychologist, or other team member participates in the group as a facilitator of this process.

Siblings of children with spina bifida can also benefit from specialized programs (Featherstone, 1980; Pinyerd, 1983). Brothers and sisters are particularly vulnerable when the care of the handicapped child absorbs a disproportionate amount of parental time and energy. Expectations and demands on the sibling may be excessive, resulting in such acting-out behaviors as wetting, soiling, and poor school performance, and in behavior problems (Murphy, 1982). Sibling activity programs (and, in some cases, individual therapy) can be useful in assisting these children to increase their understanding and adjustment.

Grandparents also have special needs when a child with a physical disability is born into the family (Berns, 1980). However, parents are often too overwhelmed to deal with the emotional and informational needs of the grandparents. As a result, grandparents may be poorly informed or may have misconceptions regarding the nature of the disability. One grandmother believed that the child's shunt was placed at the back of the throat and so, she was fearful of feeding the child. In other cases, grandparents may believe that the child will "get well" with time. One mother reported that the child's grandmother repeatedly asks, "Is he still handicapped?"

In order to meet this informational need, as well as to provide emotional support, group intervention with grandparents can be offered on a regular or periodic basis. Such assistance can be provided in a discussion group or in a recreational format. Grandparents and the child with spina bifida can experience planned recreational activities that foster interpersonal understanding and interaction. This model has the added benefit of affording the parents some free time away from child care responsibilities.

In addition to these groups, routinely scheduled information-oriented programs can benefit family members. Topics of interest vary according to the ages of the children and the current issues facing the families. For example, parents of infants may wish to have information related to the nature of spina bifida and its impact on development, whereas parents of older children may have an interest in techniques for behavior management. Community resources such as social services, financial aid, day care, educational programs, and recreational opportunities can also be discussed.

Counseling Services for the Parents While many families have strong coping skills and a remarkable resilience to stress, there may be periods when they experience more stress than they have resources to manage. Other families may have had inadequate resources or maladaptive coping behaviors even before the birth of their child with myelomeningocele. These families may require individual intervention beyond the scope of the usual supportive services. Although every family has a unique reaction to the birth of an infant with a disability, sometimes a particular maladaptive response or child-rearing pattern can be identified. Extreme overprotection, rejection, or denial are examples of such behaviors. In these cases, individual counseling can assist family members in acquiring more adaptive behaviors.

Overprotection It is crucial that children be given the opportunity to explore the full extent of their skills in order to acquire a sense of self-mastery. But some parents assume excessive control over many areas of the child's life—either because of a lack of knowledge regarding the child's true abilities or to meet personal psychological needs. If a parent's overprotectiveness is a result of inadequate understanding of the child's capabilities, intervention is geared toward increasing awareness of the child's competence and strengths.

When overprotection results from the parent's psychological requirement to be needed, intervention is more complex. Counseling may be indicated to assist the parent in coping with his or her own emotional need to overprotect the child. At the same time, intervention assists the parent in managing the child in ways that will foster independent behavior. Unless this issue is addressed, the child may not progress toward independence regardless of the intensity of the therapeutic and educational program because the parent has a vested interest in maintaining the child's dependence. School entrance is especially difficult, since it decreases the parent's control over the child. The teacher and other professionals may be seen as a threat to the parent's authority, and they may have difficulty enlisting parental cooperation in carrying out the educational plan.

Overprotection can also be a manifestation of guilt related to the disability or compensation for feelings of rejection toward the child. In each of these cases, intervention involves facilitating recognition of these feelings and developing more adaptive responses. The nature of the counseling is determined by an accurate assessment of the underlying reasons for the overprotectiveness. Tew, Payne, and Laurence (1974) have documented the impact that results from the family's focusing all activities around the child with spina bifida. In their study, this pattern led to egocentricity and extreme dependence in the child, and to psychiatric symptoms in other family members.

Rejection As noted, rejection—the parent's inability to accept the child—may take the form of compensatory overprotection. At other times, rejection may be manifested as indifference or anger. Parental indifference may result from disruption in the bonding process, possibly associated with separation from the infant for medical care after birth. In other cases, the parent may maintain an emotional distance in anticipation of future separations such as institutionalization, adoption, or death. Some parents have difficulty interpreting the child's signals, which are mistakenly viewed as rejecting. Therefore, parental alienation may be in response to a perceived rejection by the child.

Hostility toward the child may arise from the multitude of pressures that the child represents, such as emotional and financial strain. Counseling is directed toward helping the parent recognize and work through these feelings. In addition, intervention involves linking the parent to supportive services. This assistance may include respite care, financial aid, visiting nurses services, and transportation support as well as home-based intervention programs. Alternative living arrangements such as foster care, adoption, or institutionalization may ultimately need to be explored.

Denial It is relatively rare that a parent completely denies the child's disability. More commonly, a parent will deny the extent or implications of the disability. For example, a parent may acknowledge the physical disability but not the impaired cognitive functioning. Parents of children with spina bifida may be especially susceptible to this tendency, since the appearance of the "cocktail party syndrome" (hyperverbal speech) may be incorrectly attributed to accelerated intellectual development.

Denial is a normal way to protect oneself from trauma and to emphasize the favorable (Vernon, 1979). It is natural for recognition of the disability to be a slow and erratic process. The parent may fluctuate between periods of unrealistic optimism and of undue pessimism regarding the child's potential. Given this process, it is difficult to differentiate between denial and hope for the child's future. Sometimes a misdiagnosis of denial results from the professional's impatience with the natural time span needed by the parent to adjust to the disability.

Intervention is indicated, however, if the parent's denial of the handicap results in inappropriate expectations being placed on the child. The practitioner should provide an explanation of the disability and emphasize the child's capabilities. This process may need to be repeated over an extended period of time. Accurate assessment of the parent's readiness to integrate such information is critical and should be given careful consideration, since denial is functional as a defense against overwhelming anxiety. A parent showing extreme denial may require ongoing psychotherapy to decrease anxiety and strengthen adaptive functioning before being able to address information regarding the disability. However, such an extreme response appears to be very rare. For the majority of parents, intervention can focus on modifying their expectations of the child.

Psychosocial Intervention for the Child Many children with spina bifida experience a healthy emotional development. It is important, however, to be aware of the factors that can undermine this desirable outcome. There are specific areas of vulnerability that can influence the emotional adjustment of the child, beginning at the earliest stages of development. According to Erikson (1963), the initial task of infancy is that of establishing a sense of basic trust that needs will be met. When that trust is not established, problems may occur later in the child's life. If the child perceives that the world is threatening or unresponsive, coping strategies may develop that eventually become maladaptive, such as rigidity, withdrawal, or perseveration.

One area of vulnerability during the early years involves parental overconcern for the child. For example, some parents may be overly fearful of leaving the child with a sitter, or they avoid any activity that may be upsetting to the child. As a result, the child quickly learns how to control the parents. A vicious cycle develops, with the parents increasingly resentful of this confinement and the child increasingly insecure and manipulative.

The child's neuromuscular impairment may also influence emotional development. Motor activity is important in providing an outlet for normal feelings of aggression as well as for facilitating initial attempts toward independence. Likewise, children during the early childhood years take great pride and interest in the control of their bodily functions, as in toilet training. The child with myelomeningocele may have limited means of mobility to pursue self-initiated exploration. Incontinence may further lessen the child's sense of self-mastery and may reinforce dependence on adults.

Peer interaction can also cause difficulties, as social experiences become increasingly important for emotional development. Social, interactive play normally assists the child in managing anxiety and fears, as well as providing an opportunity to learn imitative behaviors. This experience may be unavailable to the child with a disability if isolation from peers is prevalent.

Because of these vulnerabilities, some children with spina bifida may begin to exhibit evidence of emotional maladjustment. In such cases, professional intervention is indicated through individual, family, or group therapy. Play therapy can provide a medium for the child to resolve areas of conflict and progress toward higher levels of psychological development. For the older child, discussion and activity groups can be helpful, particularly to facilitate skills in social interaction with peers. Short-term intervention with the family to solve specific behavioral problems is another effective strategy.

Children with myelomeningocele and their families, like all other families, exhibit the whole range of coping capabilities. Effective intervention recognizes and builds from these individual differences.

CHAPTER 2

Factors
Influencing Learning

THERE ARE MANY AREAS OF EARLY DEVELOPMENT THAT NEED TO MATURE AND be integrated to form a foundation for learning. Consequently, it is important for individuals working with young children with spina bifida to be aware of how each developmental area affects the ability to learn.

In which developmental areas do some children with myelomeningocele exhibit problems? The most obvious problem is the lesion on the back, often causing paralysis below it. Any type of motor deficit usually limits, or at least delays, the independent mobility and the manipulative skills of the child. These motor skills are crucial to exploration, which, in turn, is so important to the early sensorimotor schemes from which basic perceptual and cognitive skills develop.

In addition to the lesion, there may be other problems—of the type that are frequently associated with hydrocephalus. These problems, which result from impaired neurological processing, must be addressed because they tend to have an even greater impact on the child's learning potential than the physical impairment itself.

Research has identified several areas that may interfere with the learning process in some children with myelomeningocele. They include: lack of mobility, attention deficits, visual impairments, poor arm and hand function, visual-perceptual difficulties, specific learning disabilities, and auditory-language problems. In addition, there are other factors, specifically in the area of sensory development, that have been found to influence learning. These "sensory-based" problems are related to two main areas: sensory dis-organization, which manifests itself in defensive behaviors (usually in response to tactile, movement, and auditory input); and the impaired sensory integration that may result in inefficient motor planning and bilateral integration.

Young children with myelomeningocele vary tremendously in their abili-ties. For example, some children have minor motor involvement, whereas others have major motor handicaps. Some children are intellectually gifted, whereas others have learning disabilities. Since each child with spina bifida is unique, the following discussion varies in its relevance to any specific child. One cannot assume that a particular child has difficulties in the domains that are presented. Indeed, many of these domains may be areas of strength for a specific child. Because of this variability among children, it is important to evaluate and monitor each domain in order to ensure a comprehensive, personalized program that is relevant to the individual. This chapter discusses the following: mobility, attention, vision, arm and hand function, sensory processing, visual perceptual-motor skills, intellectual abilities, and speech and language abilities.

MOBILITY

Learning is based in large part on sensorimotor experiences. It is through movement, and the sensory feedback of movement, that one learns about oneself, the environment, and the relationship of self to the environment. Sensorimotor exploration forms an important foundation for the development not only of motor skills but also of perceptual, visual-motor, language, and social-emotional skills as well. Any limitations to interaction with the environment—through deficient sensory reception, lack of mobility, or impaired manipulation—may inhibit a child's early perceptual development and thereby possibly limit his or her future intellectual capabilities.

Early communication, too, is through gestures and movement. Thus, impaired motor skills may interfere with the child's initial attempts at communication. In this way, not only language skills are inhibited but possibly social and emotional skills as well. Since movement enables a child to function independently of a caregiver, lack of movement may cause a child to remain emotionally as well as physically dependent.

Impaired mobility presents a formidable problem in itself. Yet its effects on a child's adaptive skills must also be considered in order to realize the full impact that mobility has on all of a child's functional and learning capabilities.

ATTENTION

It is commonly found that some children with myelomeningocele, particularly when associated with hydrocephalus, display both a short attention span and a high degree of distractibility. These deficit behaviors are obviously detrimental to the child's ability to concentrate and learn. Attention deficits may be a direct result of poor neurological functioning, or they may be related to the quality of environmental stimulation.

As the brain matures, it develops the capacity to screen out (inhibit) unimportant information and attend to what is necessary or important. In some children with spina bifida, the inhibitory capacity may not develop adequately;

as a result, the child is unable to attend to specific stimuli or can attend for only short periods of time. Instead, the nervous system attends to, and is distracted by, all the sensory information that it receives.

The reason that other children with spina bifida do not develop adequate attention may have to do with environmental factors. For example, if a child is given toys that are not suited to his or her developmental level—taking into account motor or perceptual problems—the presented activity will be of little interest and will not promote the child's ability to attend. Since a child's attention may increase or decrease depending on the extent to which he or she is interested or challenged, it is important to provide the child with appropriate playthings in order to stimulate not only manipulative and perceptual skills but attention and cognitive skills as well. However, a cluttered and chaotic environment may lead to disorganized behavior. The proper monitoring of auditory and visual stimulation in the environment promotes the child's ability to attend to relevant tasks.

Anderson and Spain (1977) have described ways to improve attention and decrease distractibility. Parental participation is crucial; parents can be assisted in how best to interact with their child. Certain behaviors in the child need to be encouraged while others should be ignored.

1. Encourage the child to listen and attend from an early age by:
   a. Telling or reading short stories. Ask the child questions about the story or have the child retell the story.
   b. Encouraging the child to remain "on task" for specific periods of time.
   c. Ignoring irrelevant chatter about things not related to the activity.
   d. Refocusing attention on the task at hand, with such statements as "Let's go on with what we're doing."
2. Structure the environment in such a way as to eliminate distractors. Present and remove toys appropriately. Reduce extraneous visual or auditory stimuli.
3. Present toys that will enable the child to experience success and satisfaction. When play at a higher level is being encouraged, social rewards are especially important so as to maintain the child's interest and motivation.
4. Make sure that toys are pleasurable, so that they will motivate the child's attention.

VISION

Vision is one of the first senses an infant uses to gain information about the environment. Impairments in this sense organ or in the processing of visual information can interfere with the acquisition of many skills. Some children with spina bifida may have ocular and visual difficulties. Examination by an ophthalmologist or optometrist is important to identify deficits in visual acuity such as farsightedness (hyperopia) or nearsightedness (myopia). These refractive errors can be corrected by eyeglasses. Two less common visual difficulties are strabismus and nystagmus.

Strabismus

The visual defect of strabismus is due to a muscle imbalance that causes the two eyes to be directed to different points when looking at an object in space. The eye may deviate inward (esotropia) or outward (exotropia). Since the deviation usually causes double vision and vision confusion, there is suppression of the input from the deviating eye. When suppression becomes a habit, vision in the weaker eye is gradually lost or fails to develop properly. For children who develop strabismus in the first year of life, this suppression can be very serious, since they may never develop the binocular vision that is normally established by 6 months of age. Some children have alternating strabismus in which the deviation varies between one eye and then the other.

Judgments of distance, size, and direction are facilitated by binocular vision. Although the exact effects of strabismus on the perception of spatial relations are not completely known, clinically one sees children with strabismus making errors in visual judgments during such activities as reaching and catching. The condition appears to be related to the child's inability to perceive accurately the distance between self and object.

Binocular vision influences other visual abilities, too, such as tracking and scanning—abilities that aid the child in achieving a visual understanding of spatial relationships. Later, these skills become crucial for reading and copying. In addition, object permanence, an early cognitive skill, may be delayed in a child who cannot track objects to their point of disappearance. Thus, lack of binocularity can impede cognitive skills as well as spatial perception.

Some children use a head tilt to compensate for the ocular malalignment. They position the head to accommodate for the muscular imbalance of one eye in order to improve their functional vision (Langley, 1980). If one eye deviates in, the face is often turned toward the affected side with the chin lowered. If one eye deviates out, the face is often turned toward the unaffected side with the chin raised. Another frequent observation is that a child with exotropia may be sensitive to bright light.

There are several approaches to the treatment of strabismus. The most common methods are:

1. Surgery to realign the ocular muscles
2. Patching or blurring (through eyedrops) the stronger eye, to stimulate use of the weaker eye
3. Use of prism glasses, which bend the light into the deviating eye so that there is binocular fusion
2. Binocular training performed by an optometrist

Nystagmus

In this case, the term "nystagmus" is used to describe abnormal rhythmic jerking or tremorlike movements of the eyes, usually in the horizontal plane. The condition may result from significantly reduced vision, or it may be congenital. It may diminish acuity, because the movement of the eyes decreases the information received by the macula, which is responsible for detail in the center of the visual field. The child may try to compensate for this extraneous eye movement with head nodding, head turning, or head tilting. The child may resort to posturing of the head in order to place the eyes in a position of least nystagmoid movement (called the "null point"); with nystagmus thus decreased, acuity temporarily improves.

ARM AND HAND FUNCTION

Lower extremity impairment is expected in children with spina bifida; but it is not unusual to find reduced control of the upper limbs as well. Studies have documented that a proportion of children with myelomeningocele and hydrocephalus have impaired strength, poor eye-hand coordination and manipulative abilities, reduced reaction time, and even poor tactile perception in the upper limbs (Grimm, 1976; Nelson, Saffer, Kling, & Lewinter, 1984; Prigatano, Zeiner, Pollay, & Kaplan, 1983; Sand, Taylor, Hill, Kosky, & Rawlings, 1974).

These problems are apparently present from an early age. In her longitudinal studies of children with spina bifida, Spain (1974) found eye-hand coordination difficulties present at 1 year of age that become more marked by age 3. She also identified visual defects such as strabismus and poor acuity as factors contributing to poor performance in manipulative tasks.

It is also common to find that children with higher-level lesions (above thoracic nerves 10–12) have more impaired hand function than those with lower lesions. Yet this generalization cannot be based on lesion level alone. The functional performance of children with higher lesions is influenced by a greater incidence of hydrocephalus and by more severe motor restriction than are found among children with lower lesions. Moreover, children with decreased intellectual abilities also have a higher incidence of poor hand use.

There are three major physical reasons for impaired hand function.

1. Cerebellar damage due to the Arnold-Chiari malformation can cause cerebellar ataxia, which results in problems controlling the force, rate, and range of voluntary movement. Associated difficulties include muscle weakness that is secondary to low muscle tone, poor initiation and cessation of movements, and tremors.
2. Malformation of the spine above the lesion ("cord cavitation") can cause either sensory or motor disturbances in the upper extremities.

3. Hydrocephalus may cause cell damage in the motor cortex, thus affecting not only the lower but the upper limbs as well (see Chapter 4). In such cases, the child may show pyramidal tract abnormalities such as spasticity. The presence of spasticity in the arms is a major impediment to the development of functional independence in activities of daily living.

In addition to these organic problems, there are other reasons why a child with spina bifida may not develop adequate hand function. They include the following:

1. There may be a reduced opportunity for appropriate sensory and movement experiences as a consequence of frequent hospitalizations. For example, restrictive positioning usually limits the child from playing in weight-bearing positions, and weight bearing is a prerequisite for developing shoulder stability. There may also be a lack of opportunity for manipulative play in hospital settings.
2. Delayed gross motor development, which may be exhibited in inadequate postural control of the head and trunk, as well as limitations in mobility, can retard upper extremity development.
3. Insufficient sitting balance, causing the child to continue to rely on one arm for support, significantly interferes with the child's ability to perform bilateral (two-handed) tasks in sitting. Continued reliance on one-handed propping may also interfere with the development of a hand preference.
4. The child may have a lack of opportunity to practice manual skills. Since gross motor deficits seem to draw more attention during infancy, fine motor and manipulative tasks may be overlooked. As a result, the child may not be provided with adequate stimulation for use of the upper extremities in reaching, grasping, and releasing objects.
5. Visual difficulties, as mentioned previously, may interfere with the development of manual dexterity.

Since upper limb and fine motor control are important to all the tasks of daily life, impairment in this area can have a great impact on the functional abilities of the child. Poor upper extremity control may contribute to reduced mobility, in that neurological abnormality (secondary to hydrocephalus) may interfere with teaching a child to walk with crutches. Poor spatial knowledge may also interfere with the child's learning of this mobility skill. Delay in developing the fine motor skills involved in reaching, grasping, and releasing interferes with the successful manipulation of objects in early learning activities such as stacking blocks, placing pegs, and stringing beads.

Poor fine motor performance may also influence such activities of daily living as self-feeding and dressing. Children with spina bifida may have an immature grasp of the spoon and poorly coordinated hand-to-mouth movements. Fasteners, especially buttons and snaps, are difficult for these children since they require fine pinch and the skilled use of both hands working together.

Handwriting is a highly refined task that demands not only adequate grasp and muscular control but also adequate skills in tactile and kinesthetic perception, visual perception of form and space, and motor planning. Some children with spina bifida have difficulty in handwriting because of inefficiencies in any one or all of these areas.

SENSORY PROCESSING

Sensory integration is the normal process that enables one to receive and interpret sensory information from the body and the environment in order to make adaptive, purposeful responses. In the words of Ayres (1979):

> Sensory integration is the process of organizing sensory inputs so that the brain produces a useful body response and also useful perceptions, emotions, and thoughts. Sensory integration sorts, orders, and eventually puts all of the individual sensory inputs together into a whole body function. When the functions of the brain are whole and balanced, body movements are highly adaptive, learning is easy, and good behavior is a natural outcome. (p. 28)

Integration takes place on many neural levels within the brain and is dependent on efficient processing at all of those levels. The structural hierarchy within the central nervous system is: spinal cord, brain stem, midbrain, and cerebral cortex. Each center is dependent on the reception of sensory input as well as the integrative capabilities of other centers. If the brain is unable to integrate sensations adequately, problems may arise in perceptual processing, emotional responses, motor coordination, and learning.

In some children with myelomeningocele, one may find sensory integrative and perceptual difficulties similar to those seen in children with other neurological impairments, such as cerebral palsy and minimal cerebral dysfunction (Balzer-Martin, 1980). These functional difficulties may be the result of actual neurological damage that interferes with skill acquisition, or they may be related to poor sensory processing. Inadequate processing of sensory information may occur as a result of limited stimulation, lack of experience, or poor neurological organization.

Proper sensory processing is important for the acquisition of all life skills. It provides the foundation for the development of motor abilities, attention span, perceptual skills, language, and appropriate emotional behavior. All of these competencies are important to successful learning and interaction with the environment. Dysfunction in sensory integration thus limits an individual's capacity for adaptive coping.

The difficulties in sensory integration to be discussed are: sensory disorganization expressed in "defensive" behaviors; inefficient motor planning; poor bilateral integration influencing coordinated use of the two sides of the body; and inadequate hemispheric specialization influencing the higher-level, lateralized skills of hand dominance, language acquisition, and visual-spatial perception.

Sensory Disorganization Expressed in Defensive Behaviors

Defensive behaviors are exaggerated, emotional responses to specific sensory stimuli. They can be seen as a hypersensitive response to sensory input, the most common being reactions to tactile, movement, and auditory stimulation. According to Knickerbocker (1980),

> hypersensitivity . . . causes too many stimuli to reach the brain with the same degree of intensity and relevancy. The central nervous system is overwhelmed, and the child overreacts. He responds to incoming stimuli . . . in a primitive, protective manner. (p. 35)

In the early years, defensiveness can interfere with mother-infant bonding and feeding, as well as disturb the foundations of sensory and perceptual development. Later, in the school years, defensiveness may not interfere directly with learning per se but may be the cause of maladaptive behaviors such as distractibility, extreme activity, or inappropriate aggressiveness. These behaviors often disrupt the learning process and limit interpersonal relationships. For example, distractibility may seriously influence the child's ability to function as part of a group in the classroom or with peers on the playground.

Tactile Defensiveness The tendency to react negatively to sensations of touch is tactile defensiveness. A tactually defensive child is sensitive to tactile input that others would hardly feel. Since the central nervous system is unable to inhibit the stimuli, the child reacts with flight (avoidance, withdrawal) or fight (anger, hostility). These behaviors are reflections of an attempt to achieve a protective state within the nervous system. This overactive protective system needs to be inhibited so as to permit discriminative skills (which give one information about oneself and the environment) to develop. If inhibition does not take place, there is likely to be a negative impact on many adaptive skills, including feeding and mouthing behaviors, activity level and attention span, tactile discriminative skills, and interpersonal skills.

Feeding and Mouthing Behaviors The face and mouth have a large number of sensory receptors. If they are hypersensitive, various problems can occur. Feeding may be a conflict between wanting and/or needing food and discomfort with touch, especially in and around the mouth. As solids are introduced, some young children become fussy eaters since they prefer foods with the least texture. They resist chewing and those foods that require it.

Likewise, they may have aversive reactions to hot or cold, accepting only foods and liquids that are at room temperature.

Decreased mouthing behaviors may also be noted. Reduced mouthing of objects may be caused by delayed hand-to-mouth skills or by hypersensitivity in the oral area. Oral exploration by the infant of hands, feet, and toys is important to the development of body awareness and tactile desensitization in and around the mouth. To reduce hypersensitivity, it is important to assist the infant in oral exploration of body parts and play objects.

Activity Level and Attention Span   Research (Ayres, 1979) has shown a correlation between tactile defensiveness and hyperactivity, both of which are thought to be related to lack of inhibition by higher-level brain centers. The tactually defensive child may move excessively to reduce discomfort with tactile sensation. This lack of habituation to touch causes the child to be distracted by irrelevant stimuli, thereby reducing attention to task and increasing hyperexcitability.

Since these behaviors are prevalent in some children with spina bifida and hydrocephalus, tactile defensiveness is an area that should be explored as a possible contributor to distractible behavior. The remediation of tactile problems may be a necessary first step in the management of attention deficits.

Tactile Discrimination   Skills in tactile discrimination may be compromised as a result of an overactive protective system. Since the child is always in a state of guarded protectiveness against touch, tactile exploration—which promotes the ability to localize and discriminate touch—may be reduced, and these skills may remain undeveloped. Poor localization of touch (finger agnosia) and poor identification of objects by touch alone (astereognosis) are typical problems found in defensive children.

Studies have documented the presence of such tactile processing problems as astereognosis and poor tactile discrimination in some children with myelomeningocele and hydrocephalus (Grimm, 1976; Sand et al., 1974). Since the development of visual perception is influenced by tactile exploration of the environment, these difficulties can indirectly interfere with the acquisition of visual-perceptual skills.

Interpersonal Relations   A child who is constantly in a protective state may respond to physical contact by pushing away (aggression) or by avoidance (withdrawal). These types of responses may be interpreted by others as willful rejection on the part of the child. Negative reactions may then set off a series of strained relationships between the child and family members or the child and friends.

The following are guidelines for working with a tactually defensive child:

1.   Do not impose tactile stimulation on the child. Allow the child to apply his or her own stimulation. Provide a variety of experiences such as rubbing with a terry cloth towel, lotions, powder, or textured materials.

2. When touching a tactually defensive child avoid light touch; use deep, firm pressure. Children are more sensitive around the face and inside of the arms. They are more wary of being touched where they cannot watch and monitor.
3. Combine touch with movement activities, such as rolling and crawling on various textures.
4. Encourage discriminatory abilities by naming or matching unseen objects, shapes, and textures. For example, the child can reach inside a sack, identify a toy by feeling, and then remove the toy to see if he or she was correct.

Movement Defensiveness   Defensiveness to movement has been divided into two types of hyperreactive responses: intolerance to movement and postural insecurity. The first is seen in response to movement itself, especially rapid movement or spinning. Children with intolerance to movement are apt to become carsick easily or to become upset on playground equipment. Postural insecurity is related to the child's fear of different antigravity positions. Ayres (1979) has noted that anxiety or distress is elicited in the child "whenever he is in a position to which he is not accustomed, or when he tries to assume such a position, or when someone else tries to control his movement or position. He is particularly threatened when other people move him" (p. 84). It is often difficult to tell these disorders apart, for they both cause excessive reactions. In this context, movement defensiveness is a problem in sensory processing and should not be confused with the natural fear of falling felt by children with a physical disability. The following reactions may be seen in children with movement defensiveness and/or postural insecurity.

If movement-defensive, the infant may become extremely irritable when carried, especially when being picked up. The child tends to be reluctant to move on his or her own and is content to sit in one place for long periods of time. The older child may be afraid of going up and down hills, stairs, or curbs. Since maintaining a set head position is critical to many of these children, they especially dislike turning their heads upside down. As these children mature, their play may be severely limited; they often become very passive and sedentary. They may engage only in table-top tasks or visual activities such as watching television. Left to themselves, these children may avoid the movement experiences that are vital to perceptual development, especially awareness of the body in space and awareness of spatial relationships.

Active movement is important in order to develop the inhibitory capacity of the brain to tolerate motion and prevent overstimulation. Without this experience, the child may become defensive to movement. Young children with spina bifida are frequently deprived of early movement stimulation because of their medical status. Later, their own limitations in independent mobility further compound the problem. Since movement defensiveness can influence emotional comfort as well as motor and perceptual development, it is important to provide early movement stimulation as well as to facilitate active movement in all planes. Of course, care must be taken that passive and active movement are encouraged only to an extent that is within the tolerance level of the individual child.

Auditory Defensiveness Defensiveness to sound can be defined as an adverse or hypersensitive reaction to auditory input. It can cause the child either to become irritable in response to certain sounds or to be auditorily distractible. This behavior is the outcome of poor modulation in the central nervous system, which limits the brain's ability to select and attend to relevant auditory stimulation. Anderson and Spain (1977) have reported that hypersensitivity to sound is common in children with spina bifida, but they cannot define the specific etiology of this phenomenon.

A child with auditory defensiveness, especially an infant, may react with hyperirritability and restlessness. These children cry at unexpected or high-pitched sounds and may even cover their ears. As they grow older, this sensitivity to sound can interfere with their ability to attend to a task.

Since some children with myelomeningocele and hydrocephalus are reported to be extremely hyperverbal, it is interesting to consider the connection one clinician has drawn between auditory defensiveness and hyperverbalization. Knickerbocker (1980) has interpreted the child's stream of verbalization as a mechanism to protect the self against auditory input. Verbalization serves to mitigate auditory stimulation over which the child has no control, and it avoids the obligation to listen to another.

Inefficient Motor Planning

Another problem that can result from inefficient sensory processing is apraxia—the inability to organize and carry out unfamiliar motor acts.

To develop new skills, a child must initially attend to the novel motor act and plan movements based on an accurate body scheme. Body scheme, or body percept, develops as a result of the integration of sensory information from successful motor experiences (especially tactile, vestibular, and proprioceptive sensations). Body scheme is an internal awareness of where one is in space and the position of the limbs in relation to each other and to the body as a whole. It provides constant input and feedback for guiding muscle action in the appropriate direction, with the correct speed and amount of force required to accomplish a motor act. As an act becomes familiar, less attention is needed to plan the necessary movements, and skills (such as reaching or dressing) become more automatic. Motor planning, then, is a critical step in learning a new skill, yet it is only as efficient as the ongoing sensory information it is receiving.

Children with a poor body scheme—the result of inefficient sensory processing—have difficulty in planning and performing many tasks. These children usually have trouble manipulating toys, tend to dislike sports or other gross motor activities, and may have great hardship in learning the necessary sequences for dressing and doing fastenings. Perceptual-motor abilities, which rely on good sensory integration, may also be impaired. This difficulty is likely to be evidenced in such activities as putting puzzles together, copying designs, and using a tool such as a spoon, crayon, or pencil.

Several studies on spina bifida have investigated how motor planning deficits may interfere with motor and visual-perceptual skills. Land (1977) has suggested that poor hand function, poor visual-perceptual skills, and poorer scores on performance tasks than on verbal tasks in IQ tests may actually be related to deficits in motor planning. Brunt (1980) has viewed the motor behavior in some children with myelomeningocele as being influenced by "constructional and gestural apraxia" as well as by inadequate bilateral integration and ataxic-like movements.

Anderson (1976) has also alluded to difficulties in motor planning, without using the term, in her analysis of handwriting problems in children with spina bifida. She has suggested that such difficulties may stem from the inadequate processing of sensory information (termed "sensory organization") and in the coordination of movements according to their intention (termed "motor organization"). Anderson has recognized not only impaired muscular function but also poor sensory processing and inadequate motor planning as influencing the ability to perform the complex task of writing.

Inadequate Bilateral Integration and Hemispheric Specialization

Bilateral integration refers to the integrated function of the two sides of the body. It results in such abilities as using the two sides together in an activity in a coordinated manner (bilateral motor coordination) and differentiating between the right and left sides. Hemispheric specialization refers to the tendency of the two hemispheres of the brain to develop major responsibility for processing and directing particular functions (e.g., language, spatial perception). Bilateral integration and hemispheric specialization are closely linked functions of the nervous system. They are interdependent and influence the development of many of the same skills. Bilateral integration is particularly influenced by the lower, brain stem level; hemispheric specialization occurs at the higher, cortical level. A lower-level deficit may often interfere with the integration needed for higher-level specialization.

Hemispheric specialization, or lateralization of functions, is necessary for the efficient processing of information by the brain. In a global way, the left hemisphere is usually responsible for language and skilled use of the right hand, while the right hemisphere has a dominant role in visual-spatial perception. For specialization to occur, the hemispheres need to communicate with the lower-level brain stem as well as with each other. If communication is not possible or is inadequate, they develop similar (instead of distinct) functions, for which they may not be well suited. For example, a child may fail to acquire hand dominance and remain equally unskilled in both hands. Or language centers may develop in both hemispheres, with neither performing an adequate job.

A child with poor bilateral integration may have difficulty coordinating activities that require the use of both hands or feet—either in symmetrical activities (such as clapping) or in reciprocal activities (such as crawling). The child may also have difficulty knowing right from left and be easily confused by directions that involve right and left. Frequently, there is a tendency to use the hand closest to the task in order to avoid crossing the body midline with an upper limb.

In some children with myelomeningocele and hydrocephalus, one finds these clinical problems, which seem related to poor bilateral integration and inadequate hemispheric specialization. The establishment of hand dominance is often delayed, and there is a high incidence of mixed dominance and left-handedness (Anderson, 1976; Lonton, 1976). Certain deficits in language and visual-perceptual skills are also noted in this population (Stephens, 1983). An anatomical basis for some of these problems is supported by brain research in spina bifida. Studies have found malformations at neural structures such as the brain stem and corpus callosum. For example, Gordon (1972) has reported brain stem lesions due to the Arnold-Chiari malformation. Miller and Sethi (1971) have found stretched and thinned corpus callosum fibers—the fibers connecting the hemispheres.

VISUAL PERCEPTUAL-MOTOR SKILLS

As previously discussed, children with spina bifida may exhibit problems in ocular-motor, fine motor, and sensory integrative skills. In addition, dysfunction in visual perception may be present. It can be assumed that a deficit in any one or a combination of these areas will interfere with tasks requiring visual perceptual-motor integration, such as preschool readiness activities and manipulative play. An impaired performance may reflect disorganization resulting directly from the neurological damage or failure of organization due to limited opportunities to explore the environment.

Children with myelomeningocele tend to score lower than normal children on tests of visual perception and perceptual-motor integration, particularly in the presence of hydrocephalus, with or without shunts (Lauder, Kanthor, Myers, & Resnick, 1979; McLone, Czyzewski, Raimondi, & Sommers, 1982; Soare & Raimondi, 1977; Tew & Laurence, 1975). Specific deficits are found in spatial judgment, figure-ground discrimination, visual attention to task, and eye-hand coordination. Children with lesions located lower on the spinal cord tend to exhibit better visual-perceptual test scores than do children with high lesions. This finding correlates with the fact that children with higher spinal cord lesions are more apt to have the Arnold-Chiari malformation and hydrocephalus, which are often associated with perceptual dysfunction.

Behavior observations of children with spina bifida during testing situations provides additional information. Spain (1974) has noted that in a task requiring the selection of one abstract design from a card containing the test figure plus four similar designs, many children with shunts are not able to accomplish the task within the time limit. Dodds (1975) has reported that children with hydrocephalus usually lose points on block design tests because of their slowness in trying to complete the design rather than because of errors in misplacing blocks. Another study found that the impulsivity in these children undermines their performance on tests requiring visual perception (Anderson, 1975). In addition, the children may quickly forget the instructions after beginning the activity or become confused in sequencing the steps of the task for successful completion.

In many of the studies, it is difficult to determine the specific reason for a depressed test score. The impaired performance could be related to test anxiety, attention deficits, problems in visual acuity, slow reaction time, motor incoordination, cognitive limitations, or actual perceptual dysfunction. Therefore, the results of formal testing in the area of visual perceptual-motor skills must be carefully analyzed in order to ensure an accurate interpretation of the findings.

INTELLECTUAL ABILITIES

Research has suggested that children with myelomeningocele, particularly those children with hydrocephalus, tend to score lower on intelligence tests than nonhandicapped children (Hunt & Holmes, 1976; Shurtleff, Flotz, & Loeser, 1973). In general, the children with shunted hydrocephalus achieve higher verbal than performance scores.

It is important to remember, however, that the majority of children with myelomeningocele have normal intelligence (Soare & Raimondi, 1977). A study by McLone and his associates (1982) has reported IQ scores in the average range for children without hydrocephalus and for children with shunted hydrocephalus but no history of central nervous system infection. It appears that intellectual function is most compromised if the child with myelomeningocele and shunted hydrocephalus has experienced infection of the ventricular system and/or meninges.

Some children with myelomeningocele (particularly those with high lesions and hydrocephalus) have selective cognitive deficits that may appropriately be considered learning disabilities (Hoffman, 1981). These discrete learning problems are increasingly receiving attention (Agness, 1983).

As measures of learning potential, intelligence tests have certain limitations. Discrete problems in visual perception, language, or fine motor control can impair a child's test performance and artificially deflate an IQ score, so that a true measure of intelligence is not achieved. Caution is in order to avoid overemphasis on the significance of IQ testing.

As just mentioned, one should not assume that a child will have intellectual impairments just because he or she has a diagnosis of myelomeningocele. Most children with neural tube defects have normal intellectual function. Lowered expectations by parents and professionals can lead to a self-fulfilling prophesy of lowered motivation and performance by the child. At present, great progress is being made in neonatal intensive care, neurosurgical procedures, and ongoing medical monitoring. Likewise, educational and therapeutic intervention is now available for children at a much earlier age. It is hoped that these positive developments will result in greater intellectual and academic achievement by today's young children.

SPEECH AND LANGUAGE ABILITIES

If one views language as a result of the child's interaction with the environment and integration of sensorimotor experience, then some children with physical disabilities may be slow in achieving the prerequisite skills for early communication. The following problems are observed in some infants and toddlers with spina bifida:

1. Delays in the developmental progression of play and manipulation of toys
2. Poor attention to moving objects
3. Failure to search for objects when out of sight (that is, failure to achieve object permanence)
4. Difficulty in imitating gestures due to cognitive or motor deficits
5. Delay in the use of gestures, vocalization, and, later, words to communicate

Older children, especially those with hydrocephalus (with or without shunts), may exhibit hyperverbal behavior—referred to as the semantic-pragmatic syndrome or the "cocktail party syndrome" (Rahlson, 1983). In these children, there is good ability to learn words and to use fluent, adultlike speech, but limitations in comprehension are noted. Conversation tends to be used as a vehicle for social contact, rather than for the exchange of ideas (Swisher & Pinsker, 1971). Children with the "cocktail party syndrome" generally find it easier to learn the form or syntax of language than the content (meaning) and use (function) of language. The incidence of this hyperverbal behavior increases with the severity of physical disability and mental retardation, and with the presence of hydrocephalus, with or without shunts (Spain, 1974; Tew, 1979; Tew & Laurence, 1975). Research by Horn, Lorch, Lorch, and Culatta (1985) has suggested that children with spina bifida and hydrocephalus are more distractible than typical children, and that this distractibility is partially responsible for their language deficits.

Since the emergence of language in these children is often viewed as a relative strength when compared to their motor abilities, irrelevant verbal responses may be fostered and sustained by the unaware adult. This extraneous verbalization tends to decrease with age, possibly as a result of a structured classroom environment and the language demands of teachers and peers.

The following behaviors, which interrupt conversation between a speaker and listener, are common attributes of children with the semantic-pragmatic syndrome:

1. Distractibility to auditory stimuli
2. Hyperverbality or continuous talking in conversation
3. Poor comprehension of vocabulary despite adequate memory of words
4. Inability to establish or maintain a topic in conversation
5. Excessive use of such social phrases as "Oh, come on!"
6. Repetition of responses that serve no function
7. Use of responses that are social or personal in nature rather than related to the topic
8. Inappropriate use of words due to inadequate comprehension
9. Difficulty using language to reason about events
10. Failure to terminate a topic with appropriate verbal or nonverbal cues

Parents and professionals should always be alert for indications of hearing impairments, articulation deficits, dysfluencies, and disorders in voice quality (Radke & Gosky, 1981). These problems in speech production occur among children in general, and the boy or girl with spina bifida is no exception.

Careful assessment of the speech and language skills of the child is important to ensure optimal development. Deviant or delayed language may impede social, intellectual, and academic progress. Language disorders may influence attention to stories, understanding of explanations, and the ability to follow directions, as well as overall functioning in the home and classroom.

SUMMARY

This chapter has enumerated specific factors influencing the learning and adaptive performance of some children with myelomeningocele. These factors include mobility, attention, vision, arm and hand function, sensory processing, visual perceptual-motor skills, intellectual abilities, and speech and language abilities. It is important that every child receive a comprehensive assessment to determine areas of strength and weakness.

Children with spina bifida differ greatly in their degree of physical involvement and the presence of associated problems. The practitioner should not prejudge the child's status or potential in any developmental domain purely on the basis of the medical diagnosis. The variability among these children warrants an individualized approach to programming. Intervention strategies are geared to remediate deficits that are amenable to change and to compensate for those that are not. Emphasis is always placed on the individual child's strengths and assets.

♦ **CHAPTER 3** ♦

Sensorimotor Assessment and Intervention

SENSORIMOTOR ASSESSMENT, PLANNING FOR SERVICES, DEVELOPMENTAL principles of intervention, and strategies to facilitate motor development are addressed in this chapter. Although the discussion focuses primarily on the functions of occupational and physical therapists, all members of the inter-disciplinary team should have basic knowledge in this area and apply such knowledge in their professional practice. Sensorimotor behavior is relevant to all aspects of the child's development.

SENSORIMOTOR ASSESSMENT

In the motor assessment of the child with myelomeningocele, the clinician is concerned both with the child's level of spinal cord lesion and with the presence of associated neuromotor deficits. A review of the child's medical and de-velopmental history is essential in determining those aspects of function that will require specific assessment. The sensorimotor evaluation should test range of motion of the joints, muscle tone, muscle strength, sensation, movement skills, postural control, and sensory integrative skills.

Range of Motion of the Joints

The orthopaedic anomalies most frequently seen in children with spina bifida include spinal deformities, unilateral or bilateral hip dislocations and sub-luxations, contractures and fractures of the legs, and foot deformities. The assessment and management of spinal curvatures, hip dislocations, and foot deformities are presented in Chapter 4.

Passive range of motion is assessed in all joints of the extremities and trunk. Excessive range of motion, frequently found in joints of the upper extremities in children with spina bifida having secondary hypotonia, is as important to record as limitations of joint range in the lower extremities. When there is marked hypermobility, particularly in the wrist and finger joints, the child may be at risk for difficulties in fine motor control owing to lack of joint stability. Limitations of joint range in the trunk and lower extremities are typically due to congenital fractures, joint anomalies, or an imbalance in the action of muscle groups (e.g., hip flexion contractures in the absence of innervation to the extensor muscles of the hip).

Spine   Range of motion of the spine should always be assessed in the infant or child with spina bifida. Cervical or neck range is evaluated by passively moving the child's head in flexion and extension (bending forward and backward), lateral flexion (side-to-side motions of the ear toward the shoulder), and rotation (turning the chin toward the shoulder). If the child is capable of understanding verbal instructions, neck and trunk range is also assessed actively, with the child performing the movements independently.

Range of motion in the upper and lower trunk is checked for flexion and extension, lateral flexion (bending sideways), and rotation (turning the shoulders in a direction opposite to that of the pelvis). Limitation of movement in any area is recorded, and determination is made as to the cause (e.g., abnormal muscle tone, skeletal or orthopaedic anomalies).

Children with spina bifida may develop spinal curvatures. The most common is a scoliosis in which the spine deviates laterally. Some curvatures can be diagnosed within the initial 2–3 years of life and are therefore termed congenital anomalies. Other children do not exhibit spinal deformities until adolescence. Regardless of the age of onset, the therapist and orthopaedic surgeon should monitor the condition closely for changes in active and passive spinal range of motion and any progression in the degree of curvature.

Hip   Range of motion at the hip joint includes flexion/extension, abduction/adduction, and internal/external rotation. Frequently, the child with myelomeningocele exhibits limitations into hip extension and abduction (i.e., movement of the leg away from the midline of the body) because of the imbalance of muscle activity in the lower extremities. As a partial result of this muscular imbalance, subluxations and dislocations of the hips are relatively common either unilaterally or bilaterally. A congenitally dislocated hip limits the range of motion into abduction.

Hip flexor tightness is often present bilaterally. The therapist can assess this tightness by using the Thomas test. The infant or child is positioned in supine lying on a table-height surface, and both lower extremities are simultaneously flexed onto the child's abdomen (knees-to-chest posture). One leg is then allowed to extend passively until it hangs off the table surface. The practitioner should be careful that the trunk does not laterally flex to compensate for any flexor tightness or contracture. The angle of tightness is determined on the side of the extended hip. One measures the position of the lower extremity in relation to the flat table surface.

Knee   The knee joint is assessed for flexion and extension. Flexor range is assessed with the child in the prone position. Extension is evaluated with the child in the supine-lying or sitting position. The knee joint also has a limited range of internal and external rotation when the knee is flexed in a non–weight-bearing position (transverse rotation).

Ankle When assessing range of motion at the ankle, the therapist records limitations of both the upper ankle joint (up and down motions of dorsiflexion and plantar flexion at the talocalcaneal joint) and the lower ankle joint (side-to-side motions of inversion and eversion at the subtalor joint). Excessive range is frequently found with dorsiflexion due to a lack of muscle innervation and resulting talocalcaneal subluxation. This factor needs to be considered when determining activities for standing and ambulation as well as requirements for braces.

Ankle muscle strength and tone are also relevant. All active, isolated movements of the ankle and toes should be recorded. The tendency to develop ankle contractures increases if there is no movement present or if muscle groups are contracting unopposed (e.g., when ankle dorsiflexion is present but active plantar flexion is absent).

The infant with spina bifida may have orthopaedic anomalies in one or both feet. The deformities are usually congenital and nontraumatic in origin and are therefore categorized as club feet. A common deformity is for the foot to be contracted into a plantar flexed and inverted position (i.e., pointed downward and turned in). However, the degree of deviation and the extent of the deformity varies from child to child.

Muscle Tone

Muscle tone is assessed throughout the body. Abnormal tone may be present above and below the level of lesion when there are associated neuromotor deficits resulting from hydrocephalus and upper motor neuron involvement. Muscle tone is evaluated in response to passive movement of the limbs and trunk, and through observation of the child's movement patterns. A degree of hypotonia in the upper extremities and trunk is common in many children with spina bifida. Muscle tone may also be increased above or below the level of lesion, depending on the type and extent of cortical involvement. Spasticity is prevalent in the upper and/or lower extremities of some children. The therapist is alerted to the occasional presence of asymmetries in muscle tone in the trunk and limbs, indicating that one side of the body is more affected than the other side. The assessment of children with central nervous system deficits has been discussed in detail by Bly (1983), Molnar (1985), and Scherzer and Tscharnuter (1982).

Muscle Strength

When muscle tone is normal, a manual muscle test may be utilized to determine the specific strength of muscle groups in the trunk and extremities. In the presence of hypotonia or hypertonicity (spasticity), accurate muscle testing is not possible. In this case, the child's ability to perform antigravity movements can be indirectly evaluated by observation of movement patterns and performance in the tasks of daily living.

DeSouza and Carroll (1976) have categorized individuals with myelomeningocele into four groups, based on the level of the neurosegmental lesion: thoracic, upper lumbar, lower lumbar, and sacral. A lesion at the thoracic level indicates no power in the muscles crossing the hip joint or distal to it. In a lesion at the upper lumbar level, there may be some muscle power in the hip flexors or adductors and in the extensors of the knee. In a lesion at the lower lumbar level, some muscle activity may be seen in the hip abductors, knee flexors, and ankle dorsiflexors. In a sacral lesion, power may be present in the hip extensors and plantar flexors of the ankle and toes.

Sensation

Pain, temperature, and touch are assessed in the extremities and trunk in relation to dermatomal innervation. Due to the distribution pattern of the nerve supply to the body, a deficit in the sensory or motor status can identify which spinal nerves are damaged (see Appendix A). In general, a lesion at the thoracic level results in no sensation below the hips, whereas an upper lumbar lesion allows some sensation below the hips. Frequently in lower lumbar and sacral lesions, the sensory and motor levels are not consistent. In very young children, this sensory assessment is usually conducted in an informal manner. The examiner closely observes any change in the child's behavior in response to the stimulation.

In assessing sensation in the upper extremities, one should look for possible disorders in sensory processing, such as poor tactile and kinesthetic discrimination, astereognosis, and defensive reactions to touch or movement. Information regarding sensation in the legs is important for planning intervention and for instructing the child and parent in safety precautions and skin care.

Movement Skills

Standardized developmental scales and informal motor assessment batteries may be helpful initially in providing a frame of reference for observing the functional and motor capabilities of the child. These tools may be useful in developing broad intervention goals based on the normal developmental sequence. However, several factors need to be considered when standardized tests are applied to children with physical handicaps.

First, developmental scales provide a quantitative measure of a child's motor performance with minimal criteria for judging the quality of movement. One needs to be concerned not only with the accomplishment of a motor milestone but also with the qualitative manner in which the child performs the task. Second, age norms for specific motor abilities are usually based on the average age level of accomplishment. That is, the stated age level reflects the time when approximately half of all children are expected to demonstrate the specific motor skill. Therefore, one should view the age norms cautiously in order to avoid overinterpretation of their significance; there is great variability in the age at which children achieve developmental milestones. Finally, in applying standardized tests, the clinician needs to be aware that developmental stages overlap and that some children may even skip stages. In interpreting results from motor scales, attention is required to analyze the impact of neuromotor deficits on performance. The important issue is how and why the child can do some motor tasks but not others. A test score does not provide these answers.

Observation of the quality of movement skills is of primary importance in developing goals and determining the frequency of therapy sessions. In observing the child's motor control in stable positions and in transitional movement between positions (e.g., progressing from prone lying up to standing, if possible), the therapist analyzes the extent to which components of movement patterns are mature, primitive, or abnormal.

Primitive Patterns Primitive patterns are those movements seen in normal early development for a period of time. However, they may persist in the older child beyond the expected chronological age. An example of a primitive movement in the normal child is an early sitting and walking pattern in which the arms are held in a "high guard" position to assist the child in balancing (e.g., hands over the head to stabilize the trunk). The child with myelomeningocele may persist in using this primitive pattern at a later age to compensate for poor trunk control in sitting.

Other primitive patterns that may be seen in the infant and young child with spina bifida include persistent reaching with a pronated forearm (palm of the hand always down) and use of a raking-type grasp with the fingers (picking up an object with a gross scraping of the hand instead of pinch patterns). In gross motor skills, primitive positioning of the shoulder in internal rotation may persist during weight bearing in the quadrupedal (all-fours) position or in ambulation with crutches.

Abnormal Patterns Abnormal movement patterns are those not observed in normal development at any time. Examples include maintaining the hands persistently in a fisted position, opisthotonos (marked arching of the body into extension), unilateral responses in the parachute or Moro reactions (only one arm responds in testing), or the presence of an obligatory asymmetrical tonic neck reflex (Fiorentino, 1981). This latter reflex is seen in normal infants under 4 months of age before it is later modified and integrated during maturation. The asymmetrical tonic neck reflex is elicited by a turn of the head resulting in an increase of extensor muscle tone on the side the face is turned toward and an increase of flexion tone on the skull side (the opposite side). Under 4 months of age, the infant may temporarily assume a "fencing" position (extension of limbs on the face side and flexion of the limbs on the skull side). However, the influence of this reflex should never be dominant, even in the young infant.

In planning the intervention program, it is important to make a distinction between abnormal patterns of movement that will have negative effects on development, and compensatory movements that the child utilizes in order to function. In many cases, use of compensatory patterns is a necessity for mobility and as such should not be discouraged. Reliance on the arms in pushing to sitting is a typical example of a functional compensatory pattern. In a child with a high-level lesion, this pattern would be emphasized in the therapy program. It is in cases where the movement pattern hinders further development in the child that intervention focuses on inhibiting and altering the pattern. For example, reaching with the arms can be impaired by habitual use of strong scapular adduction (pulling the shoulder blades together). In such cases, the habitual pattern of scapular adduction would be modified in therapy to prevent its negative impact on functional use of the arms.

Postural Control

Assessment of postural control includes observation of the development of proximal stability, postural reactions (such as head and trunk righting reactions and equilibrium reactions), and the extent to which primitive tonic reflexes have been integrated.

Essential to the child's achievement of postural control in the trunk is the development of proximal stability in the shoulder and pelvic areas. Normally, proximal control of the scapulae and pelvis allows the child to assume and maintain certain positions (such as prone-on-elbows, sitting, and standing) and provides a stable base for distal movement of the limbs. If there is hypotonia, shoulder girdle instability may be demonstrated by scapular winging or an excess of scapular movement on the chest wall. Scapular winging is most obvious during weight bearing on the upper extremities, but it is also observable during forward reach. The scapula does not maintain a secure position against the rib cage but instead protrudes out under the skin. (One can readily observe the medial border and inferior angle of the scapula jutting from the back.) In the child with spina bifida, developing scapular stability is an important prerequisite for use of the arms and is also a factor in determining the child's potential for independent mobility in self-initiated rolling, belly crawling, wheelchair mobility, and ambulation.

Pelvic stability is frequently insufficient in the child on account of bony anomalies and inadequate muscle innervation. Pelvic control is usually present in anterior weight shifting, but it is lacking when the pelvis is passively tilted posteriorly owing to a lack of gluteal muscles and decreased abdominal strength. Abdominal musculature may be weak partly because of compensatory overuse of the hip flexors. Active mobility of the pelvis is generally observed in varying degrees of movement anteriorly and laterally. Posterior tilt and rotation of the pelvis (twisting motion) are usually the most impaired active movements.

Righting and equilibrium reactions are essential for maintaining an erect and adaptive posture against gravity. Righting reactions permit the child to maintain the position of the head in space and provide the ability to restore correct alignment of the head, trunk, and limbs. For example, righting reactions are seen when the child is held vertically in the adult's arms and tilted to the side. The normal response is for the head and trunk to move laterally away from the direction of tilt in order to align the head and trunk vertically in space. Righting reactions are also active in introducing rotation through the body axis, which leads to rolling. If the pelvis or shoulders are out of alignment with the trunk, the infant will unravel (derotate) and roll over. Development of righting reactions may be delayed or absent because of abnormal muscle tone or denervation of muscles below the level of lesion.

Equilibrium reactions evolve from righting reactions. Since both are balance responses, it is often difficult to tell them apart in the preschool child; and, from a functional perspective, it is probably not necessary to do so. Equilibrium reactions are elicited primarily by stimulation of the labyrinths in the inner ear and provide adaptation of the body when the center of gravity is changed through movement of the support surface or the body.

Equilibrium reactions take two forms: 1) subtle changes in muscle tone to maintain an antigravity position (e.g., postural sway), and 2) automatic compensatory movements in reaction to an abrupt displacement of the center of gravity (e.g., shift of body parts away from the direction of fall, or stepping and hopping movements to regain one's base of support). In normal development, equilibrium reactions are observed in the prone position at approximately 6 months, in supine at 7 months, in sitting at 8 months, in quadruped at 9–10 months, and in standing at 12–15 months. Most children with spina bifida demonstrate moderate deficiencies in these reactions.

Protective extension reactions are an automatic thrust of an upper extremity away from the body to protect one from falling. In normal development, protective reactions in sitting are noted in a forward direction at 6–7 months, toward the side at 7–8 months, and in a backward direction at 9–10 months. The presence of these responses is particularly important for the child with a high-level lesion, who will have to rely on arm support to maintain sitting. The child who lacks normal righting and equilibrium reactions and trunk control will be dependent on protective extension reactions for a safe sitting position.

Sensory Integrative Skills

A history of the child's sensory functioning is useful in screening for early signs of deficits in sensory processing. This information can be obtained through interviewing the parents regarding the child's responses to movement (vestibular and proprioceptive sensation), touch, and auditory stimulation (Larson, 1982; Williamson, 1981). One should try to identify which sensory channels are areas of relative strength and weakness. Are certain sensory systems hyporeactive or hyperreactive? Does the child have a major learning mode (visual, auditory, kinesthetic)? Are there specific deficits in sensory processing leading to poor bilateral integration, defensive behaviors, or problems in motor planning? Chapter 6 provides a further discussion of assessment procedures as well as interventions for sensory and perceptual dysfunction.

PLANNING FOR INTERVENTION

Based on the sensorimotor assessment, planning for intervention must consider the following issues:

1. Level of lesion and available muscle power
2. Presence of orthopaedic anomalies that affect the acquisition of motor skills
3. Muscle tone and quality of movement patterns
4. Presence and extent of sensory integrative and neurological deficits that affect motor learning

The development of realistic objectives for therapy is dependent on the combined influence of these factors on the child's motor potential. Children with the same level of lesion may have different goals of intervention, based on variations in tolerance to movement, cognitive status, abnormal muscle tone (particularly in the trunk and arms), perceptual deficits, and related concerns.

The critical therapeutic questions are: "*How* does the child perform?" and "*Why* does the child organize movements in this manner?" These are qualitative concerns that are not addressed by standardized developmental scales. A solid knowledge of the processes of normal and abnormal development is required in order to intervene effectively. Otherwise, therapy is limited to the teaching of isolated, fragmentary skills.

When planning for intervention, the clinician needs to know the underlying components of movement, the prerequisite behaviors necessary for the attainment of a new motor skill. For example, it is important to identify the movement patterns and activities in the prone and supine positions that specifically prepare the infant for independent sitting with arm support. Connor, Williamson, and Siepp (1978) have suggested analyzing each motor task according to: 1) the components of movement required to master the skill, 2) the future skills of which this act may be considered an important component, and 3) the cognitive and social abilities likely to be facilitated by this motor accomplishment.

Broad objectives of intervention should include:
1. To increase and maintain active and passive range of motion
2. To prevent contractures and deformities
3. To facilitate desired motor skills with a minimum of abnormal movement patterns
4. To foster functional independence and mobility in the environment

DEVELOPMENTAL PRINCIPLES OF INTERVENTION

Intervention draws on developmental, sensory integrative, and neurophysiological theories, integrating concepts and principles that encourage development of the total child. Therapy is founded on an understanding of the normal sequence for developing motor control. The following principles, related to the acquisition of coordinated movement in infancy, serve as guidelines in the therapeutic process:

1. Development of postural control against gravity proceeds in a cephalo-to-caudal and proximal-to-distal direction (that is, from head to feet and from the center of the body out through the limbs).
2. Development of coordinated movement begins with extensor muscle control, closely followed by flexor control. Controlled action of flexor and extensor muscles is required for lateral flexion of the head and trunk. These motor components prepare for the development of movement with rotation in a diagonal plane.
3. Functional movement develops in a predictable sequence. The newborn demonstrates uncontrolled mobility in the form of random movement of the extremities. Gradually, stable positions can be maintained, followed by the ability to weight-shift the trunk on supporting limbs. An example of this principle is the assumption of the prone-on-elbows position, followed by the ability to weight-shift in the position, and finally the ability to reach out with one arm. A similar sequence in the development of controlled weight shifting is observed in the quadruped, sitting, and standing positions. In each position, controlled weight shifting occurs in an anterior-posterior direction first, followed by weight shifting laterally (side to side), and finally weight shifting and movement in a diagonal plane with rotation. The acquisition of proximal stability, weight shifting, and control of the scapulae and pelvis allows the child to locomote in each new position. Thus, the development of controlled movement (extension, flexion, lateral movement, and rotation) occurs during weight shifting and during play in antigravity positions while supported on the extremities.
4. The gross reflexive movement patterns of the newborn become increasingly selective and voluntary as proximal skills of stability and mobility emerge in the trunk.

5. Postural control is dependent on neuromuscular reflex maturation. Primitive reflexes are gradually integrated and altered by the development of higher-level reactions of righting and equilibrium (mediated primarily at the midbrain and cortical levels).

6. Normal processing of sensory input is instrumental in the development of motor control. Sensory feedback serves a primary role in detecting errors in motor execution and in correcting them. Some motor tasks, however, are less dependent on sensory monitoring than others.

INTERVENTION STRATEGIES

The remainder of this chapter focuses on intervention strategies based on neurophysiological and neurodevelopmental approaches as they apply to children with myelomeningocele. Therapeutic handling procedures inhibit the influence of abnormal muscle tone and facilitate the development of more normal movement patterns. Knowledge of child development provides the foundation for directing and grading the therapeutic process. The head, scapulae, and pelvis are frequently used as key points of control in handling and positioning the child. (For further discussion of intervention for children with neuromotor handicaps, see Badell-Ribera [1985], Childs [1977], Farber [1982], and Scherzer & Tscharnuter [1982].)

Intervention strategies and sample activities are presented to address the following areas: head control, tolerance to movement, lower extremity positioning and sensory experiences, scapular control and upper extremity weight bearing, trunk control, the development of movement skills, and ambulation.

Head Control

By 5 months of age, the normal infant achieves good head control in the supine and prone positions. In supine lying, the head is held in the midline of the body, and there is active head and neck flexion. ("Head flexion" refers to the slight flexion or "chin tuck" that occurs at the atlanto-occipital joint, where the base of the skull rests on the first cervical vertebra of the spine. "Neck flexion" is the forward bending motion that occurs throughout the rest of the cervical spine.) In prone lying, the infant lifts the head in midline, turns to look in all directions while propping on elbows, and flexes the head and neck to look down at hands or toys. The child maintains the head in midline when held in a supported sitting position by an adult and laterally rights the head in response to changes in the center of gravity. The ability to right the head results from the combined action of flexor and extensor muscle groups.

The infant with myelomeningocele and accompanying hydrocephalus may be at risk for developing atypical or abnormal movement patterns. Early signs (birth to 4 months) of a secondary neuromotor deficit include: delayed development of head control, an excess of extensor muscle use in lifting the head, the presence of obligatory reflexes (such as the asymmetrical tonic neck reflex or the tonic labyrinthine reflex), feeding difficulties, and extreme irritability or hyperexcitability when being moved.

The presence of abnormal muscle tone (hypotonia or spasticity) has a significant effect on the course of motor development. An infant with abnormal tone predictably develops a strong predominance of extensor movement. The infant lifts the head in marked hyperextension when in the prone position. Another typical pattern is exaggerated scapular elevation and adduction as an assist in lifting the head and maintaining it in a stable position. At the same time that extensor patterns become strong, flexor skills—such as chin tucking, neck flexion, and reaching with the arms to the body midline in supine lying—are slow to develop.

With the repetition of atypical patterns, such as neck hyperextension, the infant's movement skills become stereotypic and limited. Atypical patterns that become habitual and eventually abnormal have been described as "blocks" to further development (Bly, 1983). In such cases, the development of more advanced motor skills is hindered. For example, an infant may develop marked adduction of the scapulae, which prevents assuming a good prone-on-elbows position or the ability to play with the hands together at midline in sitting. This scapular "block" interferes with the acquisition of upper extremity skills.

Early intervention in the young infant should focus on positioning and handling procedures that inhibit abnormal muscle tone, obligatory tonic reflexes, and overuse of extensor muscles while simultaneously facilitating development of the normal components of head control.

Sample Activities to Promote Head Control

A young infant can be easily handled on the lap of the practitioner who is sitting on the floor with knees bent (see Figure 3.1). The child is positioned in a supine, flexed position facing the adult. This position will inhibit a tendency toward extensor posturing of the trunk and hyperextension of the head. Toys presented below eye level encourage head flexion (a chin tuck) and possibly neck flexion. By varying the height of the knees, the adult grades the degree of head control and chin tuck required of the child. Slowly lowering the knees together or alternately provides an opportunity for early movement experiences forward and backward or side to side.

A progression of this procedure includes positioning the infant similarly on the adult's lap in side lying. This position facilitates a chin tuck and flexor control, lateral righting movements of the head, and midline play with the upper extremities (e.g., hands to mouth for exploration, hands together, and holding objects). Midline-oriented skills are prerequisites for reaching for toys and manipulating objects in space.

In the prone position, head lifting can be encouraged by stimulating the

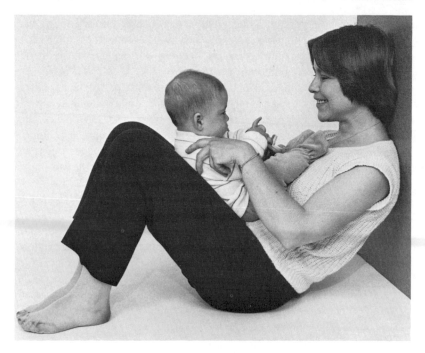

Figure 3.1. Infant held on adult's lap to promote head control.

child visually with toys. A small towel roll placed under the infant's chest may be used as additional trunk support to encourage isolated lifting of the head.

The infant with spina bifida who lacks muscle control in the pelvic and hip region may be delayed in developing normal extension against gravity in the prone position because of poor stability of the lower trunk and pelvis. In such cases, an external point of stability provided by the adult's hand on the buttocks may facilitate normal lifting of the head and assumption of the prone-on-elbows position.

Consideration should also be given to proper positioning at rest to inhibit atypical posturing and to facilitate normal head control. Overuse of supine positioning should be avoided where there is a developing predominance of extensor movement due to the influence of the tonic labyrinthine reflex. This reflex increases extensor muscle tone in the supine position (Fiorentino, 1981). Supine lying can be modified for play or napping by slightly flexing the head and neck using a small pillow, and by flexing and adducting the hips to neutral with a rolled towel or bolster as depicted in Figure 3.2. These modifications decrease the tendency to pull back into extension and encourage flexor control.

In side lying, the head should be positioned in midline (possibly resting on a pillow) and slightly flexed toward the chest. In this position, the previously noted midline skills in free play (e.g., hands together and visual regard of the hands) can be facilitated.

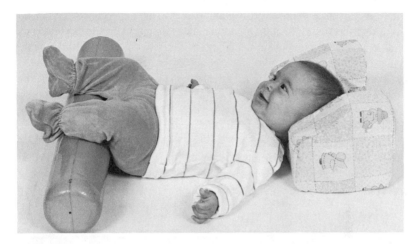

Figure 3.2.   Use of a pillow to flex head and a small bolster to flex hips in supine lying.

Prone positioning is often important to emphasize. In children who have experienced extensive postnatal hospitalization, there may be a strong resistance to lying on the abdomen and a marked preference for the supine position. This tendency can interfere with the later development of prone-lying skills, such as propping on elbows, assuming an all-fours position, and crawling. In such cases, it is advisable to increase the child's tolerance by gradually increasing the time he or she spends in the prone position. A rolled towel or small wedge positioned under the upper trunk reduces the tendency to lift the head with hyperextension. The child's arms are placed over the roll to encourage early propping on the support surface.

Techniques for proper carrying of the infant provide an opportunity to facilitate head control during daily activities. Initially, the infant can be carried in a flexed position with hips and knees bent to inhibit excessive extensor tone and encourage a midline orientation of both head and upper extremities. Carrying positions can be adopted that will foster specific therapeutic objectives. Carrying in the side-lying position, for example, encourages lateral righting reactions of the head and trunk while providing stimulation to the movement receptors (vestibular system) in a different plane. For the child who is developing spasticity, side lying is the position of choice for inhibiting muscle tone and undesired brain stem reflexes.

Tolerance to Movement

The infant with spina bifida may exhibit intolerance to movement following periods of immobility and extended hospitalization or as a symptom of neurological impairment. Intolerance to movement in the young infant may be indicated by persistent irritability, fussing, and crying in response to being moved, and an inability to be calmed with slow, rhythmic rocking by the parent. A resistance to prone positioning may also be seen. Such behaviors not only affect the infant's course of motor development but may influence the development of attachment and social interaction with the parents. Intervention emphasizes the introduction of slow, carefully graded movement experiences based on the infant's ability to integrate the sensory input and respond adaptively.

Sample Activities to Increase Tolerance to Movement

Firm, deep pressure through swaddling (shown in Figure 3.3) may be helpful as a means of comforting the irritable infant. Initially, swaddling is employed for short periods of time during stationary activities such as feeding and napping. Gradually, slow, gentle movements that are rhythmic and repetitive are

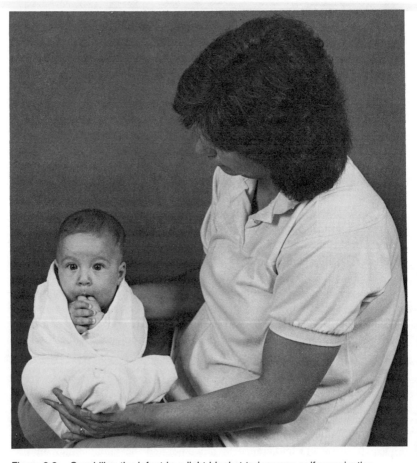

Figure 3.3. Swaddling the infant in a light blanket to increase self-organization.

introduced. While the infant is swaddled and held in a semireclining or side-lying position, the adult rocks the child forward and backward and side to side. Some infants may prefer more upright or vertical positioning during these passive movements.

Swaddling is also helpful in discouraging extensor posturing and in facilitating a midline orientation of the head and hands. However, in the presence of orthopaedic complications such as dislocated hips, swaddling of the lower extremities is usually contraindicated. Consideration can then be given to swaddling only the upper trunk and arms. It is suggested that an orthopaedic surgeon be consulted prior to utilizing swaddling techniques with children who have such complications.

In grading the sequence of intervention, it is generally easiest for the child to tolerate movement experiences while being held in a maximally supported position as the adult moves. The next progression is to move the child while he or she is being supported on the adult's lap. Finally, the child tolerates facilitation of movement on a stable surface such as the floor or a table top. It is important to note that in the older infant or toddler, self-initiated movements are generally tolerated more readily than movements superimposed by an adult's handling.

To provide movement when maximally supported, the infant is held facing forward in a flexed position close to the adult's chest. While standing, the adult weight-shifts forward and backward and side to side in a slow stepping fashion. Movement of the adult is thus translated to the infant (see Figure 3.4). The child can also be held on the lap while the adult sits on a therapy ball and moves. In these activities, the position of the child should be altered to increase tolerance in different positions, such as the prone and side-lying positions. Parents are instructed to carry the child in a variety of supported positions to provide intervention during daily caregiving.

While handling and moving the child, careful observation of the child's behavior is necessary to determine the degree of movement that the child will tolerate and the amount of external support required. Startle reactions, extensor arching of the body, and fussing may indicate that the movements are too stressful or that more postural support of the head and trunk are needed during passive movement.

In progressing to facilitation of movement on a stable surface, the adult begins by slowly weight-shifting the child in various positions. Care is taken to allow the child enough time to make normal postural adjustments to the change in posture. The long-term goal is to develop tolerance for transitional movements, such as rolling, moving from prone to sitting or from sitting to quadruped positions, and self-initiated locomotion in the environment.

The use of mobile therapy equipment, such as large vestibular boards, therapy balls, and bolsters, can be incorporated into the intervention program, depending on the child's responses. The infant may require a moderate degree

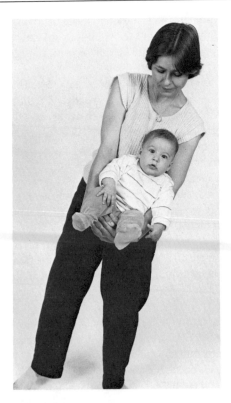

Figure 3.4. Infant held facing forward as adult weight-shifts laterally.

of external support of the trunk or pelvis by the adult. As the infant grows older, there is an increased tendency to respond adversely to such experiences if they are not self-initiated.

Intervention follows a similar course with the toddler or preschool-age child who is intolerant to movement. Therapy proceeds from providing movement experiences with the child on the adult's lap while the adult moves, to moving the child on the lap, and finally to facilitating movement in the environment. The older child, however, frequently responds more positively to self-initiated movements. Depending on the functional abilities of the child, play activities such as retrieving toys, following a rolling ball, and simple obstacle courses are used to encourage motivation to move through the environment.

Scooter boards and age-appropriate riding equipment are excellent for older children. For example, on a scooter board the child can experience moving in the prone position through space, either by pushing with the arms or by being pulled by an adult. If adequate trunk control is present, scooter board activities can also be performed in the sitting position. Whenever scooter boards are used, the child's lower extremities and feet must be sufficiently supported to prevent injury and skin breakdown due to contact with the floor. Many activities for vestibular stimulation used in the treatment of children with sensory-integrative dysfunction can be modified for the older child with spina bifida (see Ayres, 1979).

Positioning and Sensory Experiences for the Lower Extremities

Proper positioning of the lower extremities begins at birth to prevent contractures and to promote normal joint alignment and movement. Determining the proper position for the legs is dependent on the status of the hip joints, the presence of orthopaedic anomalies, and the level of lesion. The infant's orthopaedic surgeon should be consulted for contraindications in positioning, particularly in cases of dislocated hips. (See the section in Chapter 4 on therapeutic management of dislocated hips for a discussion of this topic.)

A common concern is proper positioning of the infant with active hip flexors and absent gluteal muscles who is at risk for developing hip flexion contractures. In the supine position, the legs typically rest in flexion and abduction (hips bent and away from the body midline). The child with abnormal muscle tone and resulting asymmetries in the trunk and lower extremities also requires special attention.

In prone positioning, the legs can be maintained in extension and neutral alignment by the use of bolsters made of rolled towels or Adapta foam (commercially available cylinders made of a rubberized plastic material). If there are developing asymmetries in the trunk, improved alignment can be achieved by extending the supports up the trunk. As noted in Figure 3.5, a single piece of cloth can be wrapped around each foam cylinder and secured by Velcro. Thus the cylinders maintain a secure position for the legs and do not roll to the side as the infant plays. The cloth can be readily removed for laundering.

As previously discussed, side lying is also a position of choice. The infant can be assisted to maintain the position by resting the back against the side of the crib for support, or a side-lyer can be made for the child. When holding the young infant in supported sitting, the child's legs are positioned in a neutral degree of abduction and rotation unless a hip dislocation is present. Parents should be instructed in the need for frequent changes in position to prevent skin breakdown, particularly on the feet. In addition to proper positioning, sensory stimulation of the legs is important to develop the child's body awareness and tolerance for early weight bearing.

Sample Activities to Promote Body Awareness and Modified Weight Bearing of the Lower Extremities

1. With the infant lying supine, the adult pats the feet together in foot-to-foot play as the child watches.

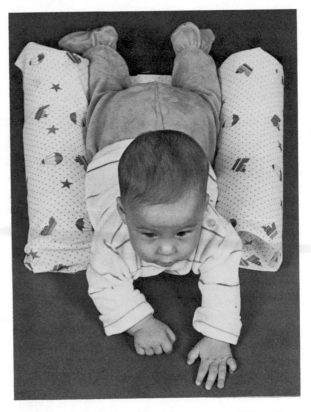

Figure 3.5. Infant in prone lying with lateral supports to maintain proper alignment.

2. The adult assists the infant to play with the legs in hand-to-knee, hand-to-foot, and foot-to-mouth patterns. When sensation is lacking in the feet, careful monitoring of the child is required during these activities to prevent injury.

3. The adult attaches ribbons or bells to the child's feet to encourage leg movements and foot play.

4. The infant faces the adult while lying supine on the lap. Modified weight bearing on the child's feet is provided by resting them against the adult's chest.

5. With the adult sitting on the floor, the child is positioned in short-sitting (standard right-angle sitting position) on the adult's thigh with the child's feet flat on the floor. With the child's legs in proper alignment, the adult exerts gentle downward pressure on the knees. The adult progresses to shifting the child's weight over the feet in forward/backward and side-to-side directions.

6. With the child in side-lying, the adult positions the upper, non–weight-bearing leg in abduction and external rotation with the foot flat on the supporting surface. The adult gently rocks the child back and forth so that weight shifts over the flat foot. The bottom leg remains in extension.
7. Diapering and bath time can be used to incorporate sensory experiences through rubbing the child with a sponge, washcloth, or towel.

Scapular Control and Weight Bearing for the Upper Extremities

By 4 months of age, the normal infant is practicing skills in proximal stability and mobility of the upper trunk and scapulae. These skills include assuming a prone position on the elbows, and shifting weight side to side from one arm to the other. In the supine position, the infant brings the hands together in midline, plucks and pulls on clothing, holds and shakes objects, and reaches hands to the knees in exploration of the body. These activities, when lying on the abdomen or back, are prerequisite skills for learning to reach with one arm in the prone-on-elbows position, for pushing up on extended arms in the prone-lying position, and for later rolling, creeping on the belly, and crawling on all fours. At the same time that the infant is developing control of the upper trunk, the lower torso and pelvis are active in providing a point of stability as a base of support.

Controlled scapular movements are essential for the development of weight bearing on the arms and for coordinated reaching and manipulation in space. An example of this critical relationship between the trunk, scapula, and humerus (upper arm) is seen in an overhead reach. As the arm moves up, the scapula follows to serve as an anchor point for supporting the extremity on the rib cage. For the reach to occur, a two-to-one ratio must exist between movement at the glenohumeral (shoulder) joint and movement of the scapula on the trunk. That is, when the arm moves 15 degrees in shoulder flexion, the glenohumeral joint contributes 10 degrees and scapular movement contributes 5 degrees. Thus, skilled use of the upper extremity is dependent on proximal stability of the scapula as it glides along the rib cage.

At this early stage of development, the infant with spina bifida and secondary hypotonia may lack the proximal control of the scapulae to achieve normal weight bearing when propped on elbows in the prone-lying position and later on extended arms. Reach patterns to the midline of the body may also be slower to develop if the acquisition of scapular stability is delayed. Figure 3.6 depicts the typical "slouching" or sagging posture of a child with hypotonia and poor scapular control when propping on the elbows.

Sample Activities to Develop Scapular Control and Weight Bearing for the Upper Extremities

Therapy focuses on inhibiting the development of atypical movement patterns resulting from abnormal muscle tone (low or high) and facilitating the action

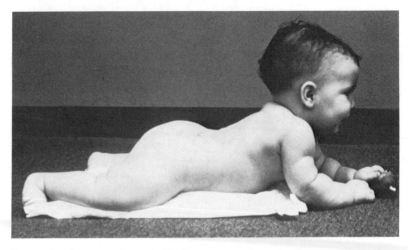

Figure 3.6. Poor scapular control in the prone-on-elbows position.

of muscles that stabilize and mobilize the scapulae in their normal range of movement. Intervention progresses developmentally in the following sequence:

1. Graded weight-bearing experiences on the upper limbs in supported positions
2. Assuming and maintaining positions in which body weight is actively supported by the child (e.g., the prone-on-elbows posture)
3. Graded weight shifting side to side and forward/backward while weight bearing
4. Controlled support on one extremity while reaching with the other

Early experiences to prepare for weight bearing should be incorporated into therapy, particularly if there is resistance to prone positioning and tactile defensiveness. Midline-oriented play, such as hands to mouth and hands together, promotes normal sensory input. Exploratory play of the body, such as rubbing hands on knees, legs, and face, is also helpful. With an older infant, tactile and kinesthetic integration is promoted by having the child pat toys or a ball with his or her palms, by assisted holding of a bottle, and by rubbing the child's hands with gentle firmness on such surfaces as a blanket, carpet, or clothing.

In daily activities, the infant can be given weight-bearing experiences on elbows or extended arms. For example, while the infant is resting semireclined supine on the adult's lap and facing the adult, the adult's chest is used as a modified weight-bearing surface as the infant reaches up with his or her hands (as well as feet). In general handling by the caregiver, the infant can be positioned in various ways to lean on one or both arms.

Initially, reaching activities to the midline in the supine position are emphasized to facilitate control of the scapulae and shoulders. Additional stability of the scapula can be provided by the adult to allow for more active reach of the arm toward objects. The adult's hand is placed on the child's upper back to keep the shoulder girdle depressed and the scapula abducted, thus promoting the reach.

In the prone-lying position, the infant is positioned on elbows with the adult's hand on the upper chest and pectoral muscles to promote active control in maintaining the position. Providing interesting toys to observe at the body midline will stimulate the child to hold the position. Later, to encourage self-initiated weight shifting, visual tracking of objects in a horizontal plane can be introduced. As the head moves to follow objects, the child's weight is shifted through the trunk.

Use of mobile surfaces, such as a large therapy ball or bolster, are helpful in developing skilled weight shifting in response to slow movements of the equipment in any direction. (Note in Figure 3.7 that the adult is keeping the child from "hanging" in the prone-on-elbows position. The shoulders are kept

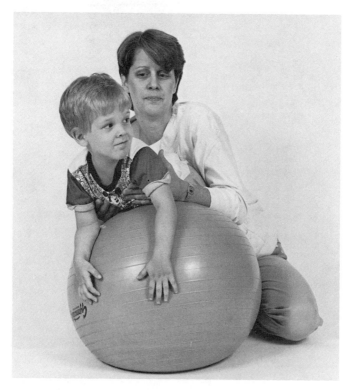

Figure 3.7. Child on therapy ball with adult controlling the weight shift.

down and the arms are aligned straight forward.) Marked elevation of the shoulders and internal rotation of the arms should be avoided. Both of these compensatory patterns will block righting reactions of the head and upper trunk.

Weight-bearing activities can also be incorporated into therapy across the adult's lap. The child is assisted to a modified side-lying position propped on one elbow and is encouraged to reach with the other arm for a toy. Self-initiated reach of the non–weight-bearing arm facilitates the experiences of holding a position (stability) and moving over the supporting arm (mobility). In this position, the practitioner can readily facilitate stabilization of the scapula with postural adjustments of the trunk by handling the scapula on the supporting side. As demonstrated in Figure 3.8, the therapist's hand is on the scapula holding it against the rib cage and preventing shoulder girdle elevation.

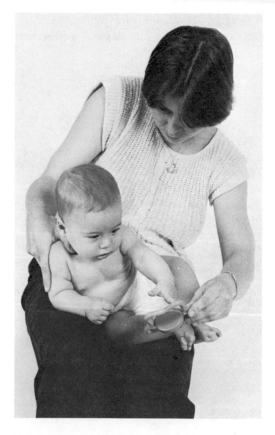

Figure 3.8.   Infant in side lying on adult's lap. Adult's hand supports the weight-bearing scapula.

To facilitate early weight bearing on extended arms, the child is positioned in the prone position over a bolster or rolled towel. Often the infant with spina bifida lacks postural reactions in the trunk to achieve normal weight shifting on extended arms. Facilitation of trunk movements by the adult will assist in promoting normal responses to movement in the upper arms. Commercially available wedges can be used to provide additional support to the trunk during weight-bearing and reaching activities in the prone position.

The toddler or preschooler may also require intervention to improve scapular stability. With the older child, weight-bearing experiences are incorporated readily during play in various positions and during movement through positions. In the floor-sitting position, propped on one arm extended to the side, the child is encouraged to reach with the other. The amount of scapular control required of the child is graded by varying the height and angle of the supporting surface and the amount of body weight supported. By varying the direction of reach, the amount of weight shifted over the supporting arm is gradually increased. For the older child, scooter board activities in the prone position can be structured at various levels of difficulty and are highly motivating. In addition, push and pull games, such as tug of war and pushing a large ball or barrel, promote stability in the upper trunk.

If the quality of weight bearing is poor, it is not unusual for protective reactions of the arms to be inefficient in the older infant and child. Without protective reactions forward, to the side, and backward, the child may be very fearful of falling. Reactions of the arms forward can be facilitated in therapy by positioning the child prone on a ball and lowering the child forward to the floor (see Figure 3.9). The speed of the forward movement is modified to elicit the reaction.

Protective extension reactions are also stimulated while the child is in the sitting position on the adult's lap, on the floor, or on a mobile surface. A shift in the child's center of gravity will elicit the arm motion to the side or backward, depending on the direction of the weight displacement. The child can be encouraged to reach behind the body in play activities, such as reaching for bubbles or a ball rolled from behind. A novel pull-toy is frequently a sufficient stimulus to encourage reaching back in a diagonal plane similar to that of a backward protective extension reaction. If undesired movement patterns such as scapular elevation and adduction are used by the child (e.g., a "high guard" position of the arms), development of protective reactions will be inhibited by the extensor posture. In this case, the child should be prepared for this higher-level skill through easier weight-bearing and reaching activities.

In the presence of normal muscle tone, other activities can be employed to develop shoulder girdle stability and weight bearing on the upper limbs. Press-ups in the sitting position increase the strength of scapular muscles, which will later be needed for crutch walking. As shown in Figure 3.10, wooden blocks are required to give the child proper leverage for the press-up.

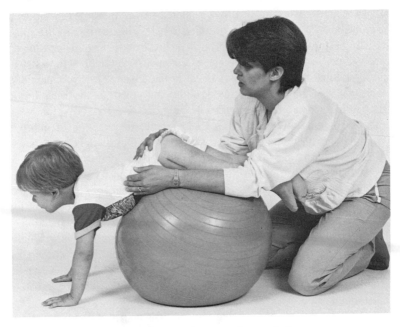

Figure 3.9. Protective extension reactions on a therapy ball.

"Scooting races" on the buttocks, wheelbarrow walking on the hands, and prone propulsion on a scooter board are other enjoyable ways to develop scapular control.

Strengthening exercises for the upper extremities can be used with discretion as long as the child does not have spasticity in the arms. It is often useful to provide resistance (manual or mechanical) to various ranges of movement as a means to promote function in transfers, self-care tasks, and mobility. Specific muscles in the upper limbs can be strengthened by progressive resistive exercises, techniques for proprioceptive neuromuscular facilitation, and isokinetic exercise.

Trunk Control

Adequate trunk control with normal postural reactions provide the basis for function in stable and mobile positions (Gilfoyle, Grady, & Moore, 1981). At approximately 5 months of age, lateral righting reactions in the trunk can be observed while holding the infant in vertical suspension and tilting the child to the side. In the prone-lying position, the infant experiences controlled lateral weight shift through the trunk with observable movements of lateral flexion. By this time, the abdominal muscles and trunk extensors work together for stability of the trunk during righting reactions and free movement. The abdominal

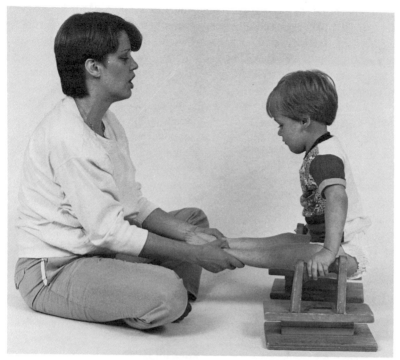

Figure 3.10. Press-ups on wooden blocks to strengthen scapular muscles.

muscles, through their action on the trunk and pelvis, influence the development of coordinated movement patterns against gravity in all positions.

Regardless of the level of lesion, it is important to determine the degree of abdominal control of the infant with myelomeningocele. In the absence of abdominal innervation, weight-shifting skills in the prone position, sitting balance, and all higher-level locomotor skills (crawling and ambulation) are affected.

When the abdominal muscles are sufficiently innervated, early intervention stresses their use in coordinated, functional patterns. If they are weak or absent, the child may exhibit atypical extension in the trunk due to muscle imbalance or the development of compensatory movement patterns. If there is potential for more abdominal use, therapy should emphasize inhibition of overactive trunk extensors and hip flexors, and facilitation of combined activity of the extensor and abdominal muscles of the trunk.

Sample Activities to Improve Trunk Control

With the young infant, activities in the supine-lying position such as chin tucking, hands to feet, and feet to mouth encourage abdominal use to stabilize the pelvis and trunk. Increased demand for abdominal control is required when the buttocks lift off the mat (posterior pelvic tilt) during foot play. As illustrated in Figure 3.11, there is active pelvic movement in "bottom lifting" and not merely hip flexion to preposition the feet for play. Activities in a semireclined position on a partially inflated therapy ball also promote early abdominal use in stabilizing the trunk.

When the child begins weight bearing on extended arms, tasks should be encouraged that stress head and neck flexion (chin tuck). The infant is presented with toys that stimulate looking down toward the hands or the supporting surface. Such activities facilitate the stabilizing action of the trunk flexors including the abdominal muscles.

Combined action of the abdominal and gluteal muscles (hip extensors) is important for the normal development of independent sitting. At approximately 6 months of age, the nonhandicapped infant maintains independent sitting with arm support, when placed. This achievement is followed by the ability to control balance in first an anterior/posterior direction, then in a lateral direction, and finally in a diagonal plane with rotation (oblique movements). These components of sitting balance emerge with the development of functional action of the trunk and hip musculature against gravity.

Many infants with spina bifida maintain sitting, when placed, within

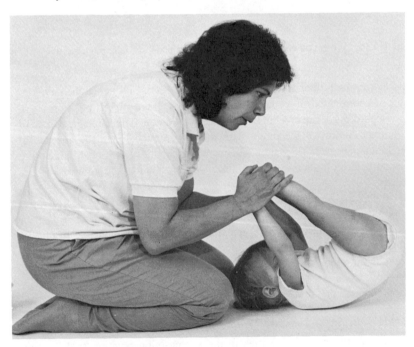

Figure 3.11. "Bottom lifting" during foot play to strengthen abdominal muscles.

normal age expectations if there are no secondary neuromotor deficits. Typically, however, normal trunk control is lacking, and postural reactions are absent. Most children tend to sit with hips maximally flexed and the pelvis tilted anteriorly, resulting in marked forward displacement of the weight (see Figure 3.12). This posture is seen in children with a variety of lesion levels and is typical of the child who has partial or absent innervation of the gluteal muscles. These hip extensors are innervated by L-4, L-5, and S-1 (spinal nerves from the fourth lumbar vertebra through the first sacral vertebra).

Sample Activities to Develop Sitting Balance

Intervention to improve sitting balance focuses on acquiring as much abdominal control as possible and developing coordinated action of the abdominal muscles and trunk extensors. For example, the child is held in the short-sitting position across the therapist's lap with the therapist's hands on the abdominal and gluteal muscles. The child's weight is displaced slightly

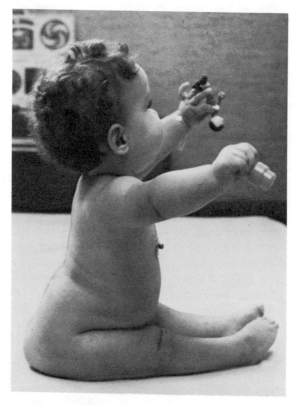

Figure 3.12.   Typical sitting position of a child with myelomeningocele.

posteriorly to facilitate action of the abdominal muscles to hold the position. As the child adjusts the trunk forward to regain an erect posture, the tendency to hyperextend the trunk and excessively flex the hips is inhibited by maintaining manual contact on the abdominal muscles. Facilitatory techniques such as tapping and stretch pressure on these muscles may be useful.

When placed in a stable floor-sitting position, the infant or toddler is encouraged to reach up for objects presented in front of him or her and above shoulder level. By reaching up to pop bubbles or swipe at a balloon, the infant experiences combined action of trunk extensors and abdominal muscles to maintain an erect trunk. Games such as "So Big" and "Pat-a-Cake" are age-appropriate means of sustaining interest. The height of reach should be graded so as to avoid compensatory hyperextension of the neck and trunk commonly observed when trunk control is poor.

To develop lateral righting reactions of the trunk, handling procedures should displace the child's weight off the body midline toward the side. This can be accomplished either by the adult weight-shifting the child from the pelvis or shoulder or by the child reaching for toys presented at the side. A manual contact by the adult on the abdominal muscles is frequently required to elicit the normal balancing response in the trunk. Figures 3.13, 3.14, and 3.15 illustrate various ways of stimulating a lateral weight shift.

The child can also face the adult while straddling the adult's lap in the sitting position. The therapist can shift the child's weight from a distal key point of control at the wrists. In this way, the therapist can easily facilitate normal lateral flexion of the head and trunk. In the same position, the adult can alternately raise and lower one leg as another means of providing an experience in lateral weight shifting.

An older child can be positioned straddling a bolster while supporting himself or herself on extended arms. Reaching activities are used to extend the trunk for erect sitting and to practice postural control in an anterior/posterior direction. Use of a high table in front of the child in this position also encourages maintaining a straight trunk during play. Therapy progresses to reaching toward the sides and rocking the bolster to elicit a lateral weight displacement.

Frequently overlooked with the toddler and older infant is the importance of controlling balance from a chair in order to reach down to the floor. To develop this skill, the child is positioned in short sitting on the adult's leg or on a bolster. Initially, the child is encouraged to reach forward, which requires graded ranges of trunk extension and hip flexion. If the gluteal muscles are absent, the child will need to rely on trunk hyperextension to return to an erect sitting position. The activity is graded by having the child reach forward to retrieve toys from footstools of varying heights.

Normally, the oblique abdominal muscles are active in rotary movements of the trunk. The upper trunk can rotate on a stable pelvis, or the pelvis can

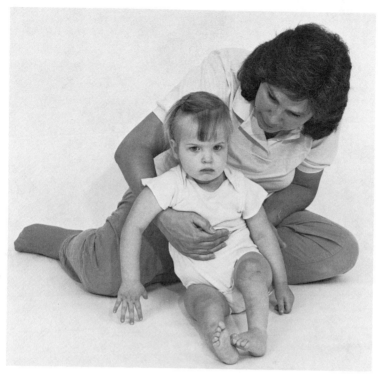

Figure 3.13. Adult weight-shifts child from the pelvis to develop lateral righting reactions of the trunk.

rotate on a stable upper trunk, as when the legs are used to initiate rolling. The internal and external oblique muscles are also important for the ability to regain balance when body weight is shifted in a diagonal plane off the midline, and for equilibrium reactions to occur. To develop rotary movements and thus facilitate activity of the oblique muscles, the adult incorporates movements with rotation in the intervention sequence. It is helpful to practice rotary patterns such as segmental rolling and movement from prone to sitting or quadruped to sitting positions. These motor tasks also improve the quality of controlled rotation of the trunk in sitting.

Often children with spina bifida may not have the muscle capacity to achieve control of pelvic rotation. However, these activities assist the children to develop whatever potential they have for lower trunk control. To enhance further the movement of the pelvis with rotation, the child is positioned in floor sitting and is encouraged to reach for toys more than an arm's length away toward the side. The child responds by supporting the body on the arm closest to the object and reaching across the body midline with the opposite arm. As the upper trunk is rotated in reaching, rotation of the pelvis follows.

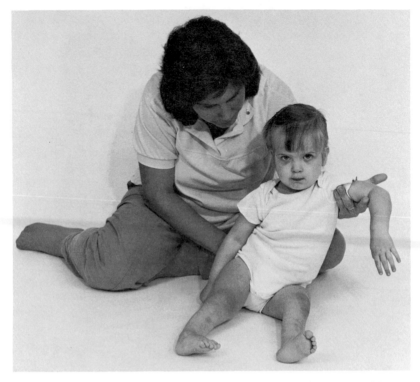

Figure 3.14. Adult weight-shifts child from the shoulder to develop lateral righting reactions of the trunk.

In sitting on the therapist's lap, with the key point of control being the pelvis, the child's weight is shifted diagonally backward to facilitate the pelvic rotation accompanying the balance reactions. The degree of posterior/diagonal weight displacement is graded depending on the child's ability to hold the position. Mobile equipment such as therapy balls and vestibular boards is appropriate for similar activities when working with the older toddler and preschool child.

The following section discusses interventions to develop rolling and skills in the prone progression, such as creeping on the belly, crawling on all fours, and transitional movement between positions.

Rolling Skills

Normal segmental rolling from supine to prone and from prone to supine positions occurs at approximately 6 months of age. Prerequisite skills for mature rolling include the presence of head and trunk righting reactions, the ability to initiate a shift in body weight, and the capacity of one segment of the

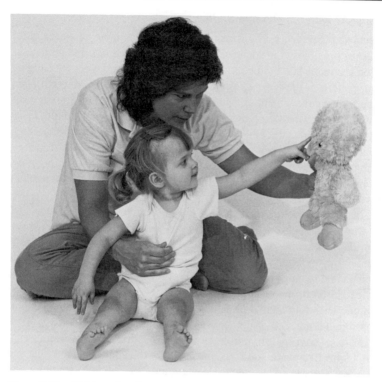

Figure 3.15. Child reaches for a toy presented by adult at the side to develop lateral righting reactions of the trunk.

trunk to rotate on the other. Normally, segmental rolling can be initiated by movement of the head, shoulder, pelvis, or leg.

Several factors may impede the infant with myelomeningocele from achieving a normal rolling pattern. Abnormal muscle tone in the upper extremities or increased extension in the supine-lying position may prevent rolling. In attempting to roll from the prone position, the child may rely on atypical patterns, such as extreme hyperextension of the head or upper trunk, to initiate the movement. Lack of muscle activity at the pelvis and hip will make weight shifting more difficult. In the latter case, the child relies exclusively on the upper extremities to roll. Dislocated hips that require positioning in maximum abduction may also make rolling impossible, as the positioning of the legs blocks the movement.

In the majority of cases, intervention emphasizes developing the prerequisites for rolling and the ability to initiate rolling from the upper trunk or shoulder. When trunk control and active pelvic movement are absent, the child is guided in developing compensatory skills to roll.

Sample Activities to Develop Rolling

Parents and caregivers are instructed in ways to facilitate as normal a rolling pattern as possible in the young child. *Rolling from the supine to prone position* can be accomplished by the infant who has active hip flexors by using a total flexor pattern of the legs. The infant first develops control through play that encourages the movement of hands to knees or feet. From this flexor position, the infant rolls to the side-lying position in a controlled sideward fall. From the side-lying position, the child is facilitated to the prone position by the adult extending the weight-bearing leg and guiding the pelvis forward toward the prone position. The child actively participates in the roll by righting the head and upper trunk. This method of rolling is the most common one for a child with active hip flexion.

In the case of a high-level lesion, the child must use the head, upper trunk, and arms to compensate for the paralyzed lower torso and legs in order to roll from the back to the abdomen. The child is taught to roll to the side-lying position by initiating with a marked swing of the arms across the body accompanied by upper trunk rotation. From the side-lying position, the child uses extension of the head and upper trunk to complete the roll to the prone position. The child should be taught to employ only the required amount of extension and not to hyperextend the head and upper trunk excessively.

Rolling from the prone to supine position first requires positioning the child's arms overhead. Assistance is given by the adult's hand on the child's abdominal muscles. This hand placement aids the pelvis in serving as a key point of control to allow the child to initiate the roll with a chin tuck. As the child flexes and rotates the neck, the adult guides the pelvis toward the side-lying position. From the side-lying position, the child lowers the body into a supine position by slowly releasing the flexor control. This technique is important, since many children will roll onto their backs by simply arching the head and upper trunk into marked extension.

In rolling from the prone-lying to supine-lying position, the tendency for the child to rely heavily on trunk extensors may be difficult to avoid. If the abdominal muscles are absent, the child has no other means but to utilize extensors in a compensatory fashion. To develop the child's optimal potential for a more normal movement pattern, the technique of assisting abdominal and pelvic control enables the child to initiate the roll with a chin tuck and neck flexion. By flexing the head and neck forward, excessive extension in the trunk is inhibited.

In developing the prerequisite skills for rolling, reaching activities across the body midline in the supine and supported sitting positions aid rotation of the upper trunk. Also, graded facilitation of weight shift in side lying on a therapy ball or lap develops the head and trunk control required during the rolling sequence. In general, working with the infant in side lying is an effective method for fostering control of movement in the midranges of the roll.

Skills in the Prone Progression

The majority of children with spina bifida achieve prone pivoting and belly crawling "commando style" regardless of their level of lesion. A child with a high-level lesion should avoid excessive weight gain, which can interfere with independent mobility. In some cases, the presence of braces may limit the child's ability to maneuver in the prone position because of the weight of the orthosis.

Prerequisite skills for belly crawling include the ability to assume the prone-on-elbows position and to shift weight from one elbow to another. Sufficient scapular stabilization and upper extremity strength are needed to pull the body weight forward. To help the child initiate belly crawling, it is useful to work on an inclined wedge with the child facing down the incline. Initially, this positioning allows gravity to assist the movement and decreases the weight the child must pull. Toys placed at the base of the incline motivate the child to move. Working on a lightweight scooter board also helps a child to develop the awareness of how arm movements can result in propelling the body forward.

Physically intact children begin to assume an all-fours (quadrupedal) position at approximately 7 months of age and achieve a reciprocal crawling pattern at 8–10 months. The ability of the child with myelomeningocele to accomplish this motor skill is dependent on the level of lesion, the presence of orthopaedic anomalies in the lower extremities, and the quality of muscle tone. While the presence of dislocated hips should not impede crawling, the quality of movement will be affected and in most cases will be difficult to improve. In general, if active hip flexion is absent, the child is limited to belly crawling, using the arms for propulsion. If hip flexion is present, the child can assume the all-fours position and crawl with varying patterns of movement, depending on the level of lesion.

In assuming the quadrupedal position, the child with spina bifida relies heavily on the upper extremities and hip flexors. Typically, the posture is maintained with marked hip flexion due to the absence of hip extensors (gluteal muscles) and insufficient abdominal use. When the child begins to crawl, there may be poor control in lateral weight shift. Consequently, the child maintains the buttocks dropped toward one side, and the legs are kept together in hip and knee flexion. The child progresses by placing the hands ahead of the body and pulling the flexed legs forward as a unit. From this position, the child tends to assume a modified side-sitting position to rest. A less common crawling pattern is similar to the "bunny hopping" seen in children with cerebral palsy. The child rests the buttocks on the floor between the heels of the feet in a "W" sitting position. Locomotion is achieved by swinging the lower torso and legs under the supporting arms in a hopping fashion.

Long-leg braces with a pelvic band provide many children with the external stability required to assume the all-fours position and to achieve mobility. At first, these children have to adjust to the additional weight of the orthosis. The crawling pattern available to them depends on the level of lesion and weight of the braces. Some children progress in the patterns previously described, whereas others may achieve a reciprocal crawl. During therapy sessions, time should be spent, in and out of the braces, practicing the movement components required in crawling.

Intervention to develop skills in quadruped emphasizes trunk control and abdominal use, stability of the pelvis, weight shifting in all directions, and achievement of as much reciprocal leg movement as possible. Specifically, most children need work on isolating hip movements on a stable pelvis to counteract the pattern of the pelvis and legs moving together as a unit. A reciprocal crawling pattern requires movements of one leg to be dissociated from movements of the other leg.

Sample Activities to Develop Skills in Quadruped

Initially, the child is positioned in quadruped over the adult's leg or a bolster. The therapist facilitates abdominal use and provides external stability at the hips to compensate for absent or weak hip extensors. As the position is maintained by the child, the therapist incorporates slow, graded rocking— forward, backward, and sideways.

The older child can exercise the abdominal muscles in an independent quadrupedal position by playing with trucks, cars, or wind-up toys. The child's body makes a bridge for the toys to move under. Using larger toys requires the child to round out the back so the toys have clearance to pass under the body. The controlled rounding of the spine is increased as the child flexes the head to see the toy underneath. When using one hand in play, the child is developing balance in a three-point supported position.

To develop asymmetrical weight bearing on the legs in quadruped, the therapist can extend one leg of the child so the body weight is supported by the other leg and hands. The child's weight is shifted slightly over the weight-bearing leg to increase isolated control at the hip.

Moving from quadruped to side-sitting and from side-sitting to quadruped is another means of working on the isolated movements of the legs that are required in crawling. Lateral weight shift in a long-sitting position on the floor (legs out straight in front of child) or in short-sitting in a chair can also be used to elicit isolated responses in the lower extremities.

The level of lesion determines the manner in which a child assumes a sitting position on the floor. When the lesion is low on the spine leaving control of the trunk intact (as with sacral lesions), the child has the ability to assume the sitting position with a normal pattern, either from supine or a variety of prone positions. Few children with thoracic lesions are able to achieve the sitting position directly from the supine position. When the lesion is between T-12 and L-1 or above, innervation of the hip flexors is absent and the child cannot assume the sitting position by moving through the quadruped position. Therefore, these children progress from the prone or supine position to the side-lying position, push up onto extended arms, and then use the arms to "walk" the body into an erect floor-sitting position. If the hip flexors are present, the children generally achieve the sitting position from the all-fours position. From the quadruped position, they typically fall into a modified side-sitting position. They may maintain this posture or reposition themselves into a long-sitting or ring-sitting position (legs in a flexed, bowed position in front of the child).

Ambulation Training

The child's ability to assume kneel-standing and standing positions without the use of braces depends on the level of lesion and the resulting motor involvement. In general, standing and ambulation should be introduced when the child is approximately 1 year of age. Learning to walk with the assistance of braces and crutches, walker, or rollator is an integral part of the program for most toddlers and preschoolers with spina bifida. Even though some of these children will give up walking as a primary means of locomotion when they become teenagers and adults because it becomes too difficult, the younger child can derive many benefits from ambulation. When ambulating, the child gains physiological benefits from being in an upright position (e.g., improved bone growth, respiration, and bladder function). Ambulation also gives the child a sense of moving from place to place in a manner similar to other children. As an exercise in itself, ambulation helps to strengthen arms and improves cardiovascular function.

In preparing the child for ambulation, the therapist should stress strengthening exercises of the arms and upper trunk through the application of manual resistance. These activities include floor-sitting press-ups, prone push-ups, and scooter board activities. With therapeutic handling, the child should move through transitional positions (from prone to quadruped to kneel-standing and back to prone). For many children, kneel-standing is an important prerequisite to standing. It can be practiced with the child's arms resting on a high table surface. The adult can facilitate the abdominal and gluteal muscles by placing the palm of his or her hands on the child at each muscle group and applying firm pressure (see Figure 3.16). This handling procedure fosters pelvic alignment toward a posterior tilt so the child does not collapse into hip flexion.

Although many children in long-leg braces with a pelvic band have been trained to ambulate using a walker or rollator by twisting at the hips to progress forward, the trend today is to begin gait training with Lofstrand (forearm) crutches and a swing-to- or swing-through gait pattern (i.e., both legs swing together to meet or go beyond the crutches). Much of the child's fear of changing from a walker or rollator to Lofstrand crutches can be avoided by introducing crutches at the initiation of the child's gait training.

Whenever possible, an attempt should be made to teach the child to stand

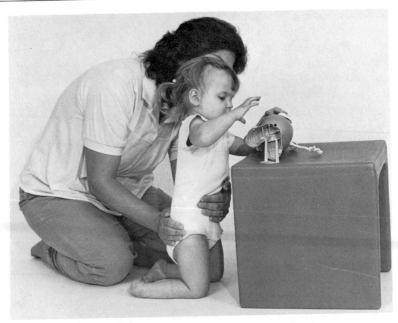

Figure 3.16. Child in kneel-standing with facilitation of abdominal and gluteal muscles by adult.

up from the floor or the wheelchair with only minimal assistance. Even a child fully braced in a long-leg orthosis with pelvic band and trunk corset can learn to take an active part in standing up rather than being passively placed in standing. As an active participant in coming to stand, the child becomes more aware of the relationship between body and space. This understanding may help decrease fear of the standing posture.

Obviously, the child with the most bracing will have the greatest difficulty in standing. However, unless hindered by lack of joint motion or marked upper extremity weakness, most children can be taught to stand up from the floor with minimal to moderate assistance.

The child with a lesion between L-1 and L-2 or below has some active hip flexion bilaterally. As a result, the child is able to assume the standing position through the quadruped and kneeling positions. As illustrated in Figures 3.17–3.21, a child with a low-level lesion achieves standing from the floor in the following manner:

1. The child begins in the prone position with the handles of the Lofstrand crutches at shoulder level and the crutch tips out in front.
2. The child pushes back into the quadruped position and takes hold of the crutches. Assistance can be given at the hips if needed. (A child with marked weakness of the arms can pull up onto a small chair instead of the

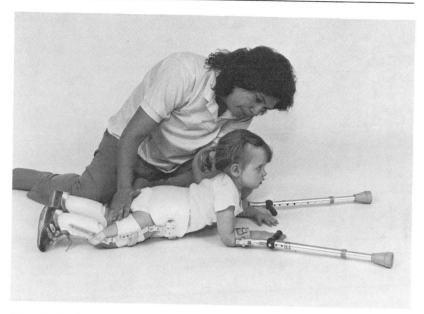

Figure 3.17. Progression from prone to standing position by child with low-level lesion. Step 1: Child is in prone position with handles of Lofstrand crutches at shoulder level and crutch tips out in front.

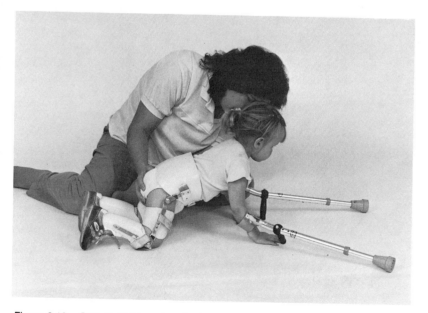

Figure 3.18. Step 2: Child pushes back into quadruped position, then takes hold of crutches.

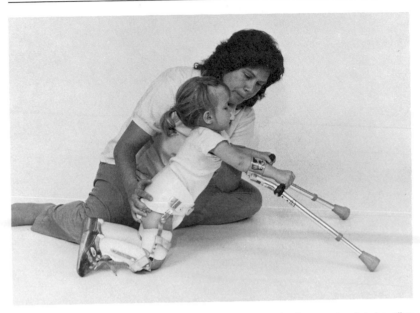

Figure 3.19. Step 3: Child places one crutch tip against the floor, pushes into kneeling position, and brings other crutch up into place.

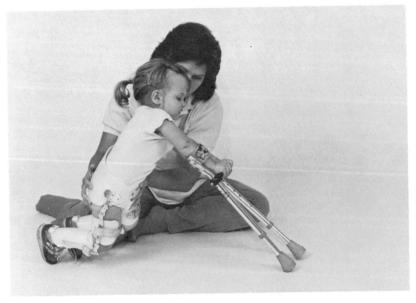

Figure 3.20. Step 4: Child pushes on both crutches to lift the knees from the floor. Knee locks on braces drop automatically once hips are behind extended, straightened knees.

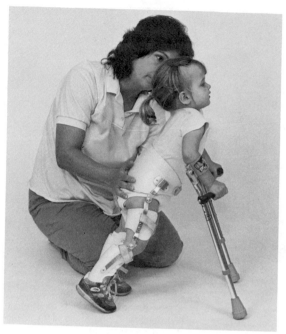

Figure 3.21.   Step 5: Child leans forward to bring hips in front of knees. Hip locks on braces drop into place once hips are straight (extended).

all-fours position. If a walker or rollator is being used instead of crutches, the child can pull up on this equipment.)

3.   By placing one crutch tip against the floor, the child pushes into a kneeling position and brings the other crutch up into place.

4.   The child pushes on both crutches in order to lift the knees from the floor. The knee locks on the braces will drop automatically once the hips are behind the extended, straight knees. Assistance can be given by pulling up and back on the pelvic band as the child pushes on the crutches.

5.   The child leans forward to bring the hips in front of the locked knees so that the hips are straight (extended). The hip locks on the braces will then drop into place. If necessary, assistance can be given at the pelvic band and the chest to help straighten the child's body into erect alignment.

The child with a lesion between T-12 and L-1 or above does not have innervation of the hip flexors. Therefore, the child cannot assume the standing position by using the quadruped and kneeling positions. Instead, this child progresses from a prone-lying to a "bear-walk" position and then achieves a standing position. In the bear-walk posture, the body weight is supported on the hands and feet. The buttocks ride high in the air since the knees are extended and the hips are flexed. As depicted in Figures 3.22–3.25, a child with a high-level lesion learns to stand from the floor in the following fashion:

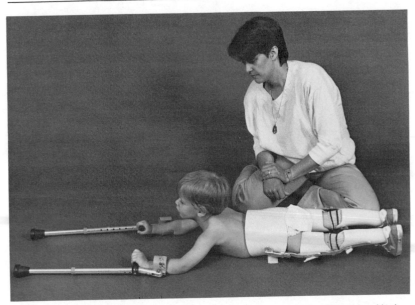

Figure 3.22. Progression from prone to standing position by child with high-level lesion. Step 1: In prone position, child locks knee joints and unlocks hip joints of braces. Lofstrand crutches are pointed straight out and child's forearms are through the cuffs.

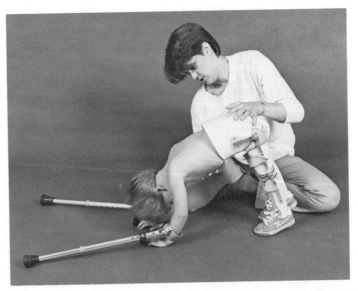

Figure 3.23. Step 2: Child pushes up on extended arms and walks on the hands back toward the feet.

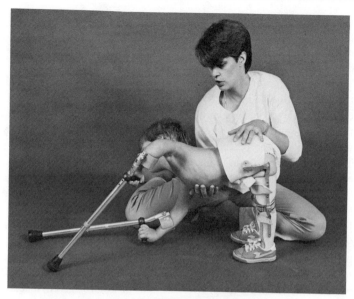

Figure 3.24.   Step 3: Child pushes up on one crutch at a time until assuming a modified bear-walk position, in which the body is supported on the feet and the two crutches.

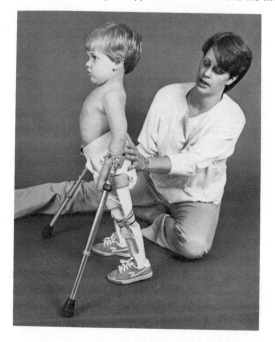

Figure 3.25.   Step 4: Child walks crutch tips backward to straighten the body over the stationary feet. When child straightens (extends) hips, drop-locks fall into place.

1. In the prone position, the child locks the knee joints of the braces and unlocks the hip joints. The Lofstrand crutches are pointed straight overhead on the floor, with the child's upper extremities through the forearm cuffs.
2. The child pushes up on extended arms and "walks" on the hands slowly back toward the feet until assuming a bear-walk position. The Lofstrand crutches passively accompany the upper extremities, since they are held by the forearm cuffs. (For the child using a walker instead of crutches, the walker can now be placed in front of the child.)
3. The child pushes up on one crutch at a time until assuming a modified bear-walk position in which the body is supported on the feet and the two crutches (the hips are still flexed). Assistance can be given by pulling up and backward on the pelvic band.
4. In order to attain erect standing, the child "walks" the crutch tips backward to straighten the body over the stationary feet. When nearly erect, the child passively straightens the hips by arching the trunk, which pushes the hips forward into extension. When the hips are straight, the drop-locks fall into position. Assistance at the pelvic band and chest can be given, if needed, to help the child assume a more upright stance.

The child who is fully braced may find it easier to stand up from the wheelchair than from the floor. This task is accomplished by the following steps (see Figures 3.26–3.28):

1. After locking the wheels of the chair, the child locks each knee joint of the braces by holding the lower leg up with one hand and pushing the lock down with the other hand.
2. Once the knees are locked, the child must turn in the chair while lowering the feet slowly to the floor. The child assumes a standing position facing the wheelchair with the hands on the armrests.
3. The child now leans forward so that the hips become extended. The drop-locks of the braces fall into place automatically when the hips are straight. The crutches are removed by the child from the crutch holder behind the chair seat. After backing away from the wheelchair, the child is ready to ambulate.

Some children may be skillful enough to assume the standing position from a wheelchair or regular chair without pivoting and transferring out backward. These children should sit forward in the chair to lock manually or positionally the knee joints of the braces. The assistive device (usually Lofstrand crutches) is appropriately placed in front of the chair. Next, the child pushes up into standing. The hip drop-locks are secured by leaning on the crutches with a forward movement of the pelvis, which causes the hips to straighten.

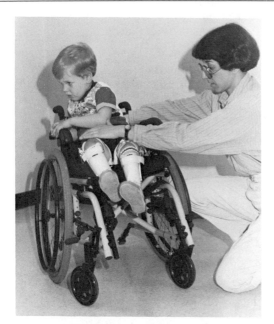

Figure 3.26. Transition from wheelchair to standing. Step 1: Child locks braces of wheelchair, then typically locks each knee joint of braces. Child then begins to turn in chair. (In this case, child safely performs the task with knee joints initially unlocked.)

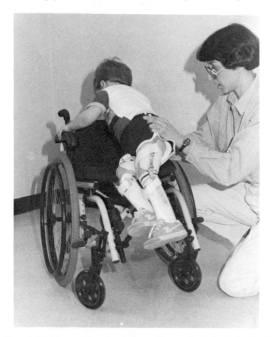

Figure 3.27. Step 2: Child must turn in chair and lower feet slowly to the floor, in order to assume standing position facing wheelchair with hands on armrests.

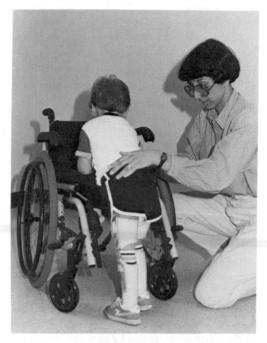

Figure 3.28. Step 3: Child leans forward so that hips become extended (straightened), and drop-locks of braces fall into place. Child then removes crutches from crutch holder behind wheelchair seat. After backing away from chair, child is ready to ambulate.

As previously mentioned, many children who are fully braced learn to ambulate with all joints locked, swinging both legs together to meet (swing-to) or go beyond (swing-through) the crutch tips. If the child has good stability at the hips and is able to bring the legs forward, ambulation may be achieved with hip joints unlocked or with long-leg braces without a pelvic band. This child may also walk with knees locked or unlocked depending on the amount of support required. A reciprocal gait pattern can then be developed.

The four-point gait is a slower pattern, but useful when teaching ambulation. The right crutch is brought forward followed by the left leg, then the left crutch is brought forward followed by the right leg. Once the child has mastered the four-point gait, change to the faster two-point gait usually occurs automatically. In the two-point gait pattern, the right crutch and left leg move together followed by the simultaneous movement of the left crutch and right leg.

If the child is able to extend the hips and knees with good strength, ambulation with short-leg braces may be possible. This child walks using a reciprocal pattern and may not need crutches if balance is good.

Sample Activities to Promote Ambulation

The child with myelomeningocele who has braces and assistive aids should be able to ambulate with little or no fear of falling. Consequently, the following gross motor activities are helpful in the development of necessary coordination.

1. Modified kick ball or soccer: The adult rolls the ball to the child, who responds by hitting the ball with a crutch, one lower extremity, or both lower extremities.
2. Modified baseball: The adult throws the ball to the child, who responds by hitting the ball with either crutch.
3. Falling practice: The child faces a foam wedge and practices falling from a standing position onto the surface. The height of the wedge is gradually decreased as the child develops confidence and proficiency.
4. Balance training: The child stands with the crutches placed approximately 10 inches in front of the body. Then the child moves the two crutches simultaneously 10 inches behind the body, without moving the feet. This shift in crutch placement is repeated numerous times. As arm strength and balance improve, the distance of placement from the child is increased.

◇ CHAPTER 4 ◇

Health Issues

IT IS IMPORTANT TO UNDERSTAND THE NEUROLOGICAL AND ORTHOPAEDIC problems of children with spina bifida and the implications for therapeutic intervention. This chapter addresses neurosurgical treatment of the lesion site and hydrocephalus, management of deformities of the spine and lower extremities, and health issues related to osteoporosis and proper skin care.

CLOSURE OF THE BACK

Neurosurgery is commonly performed in the first week of life to manage the myelomeningocele. Charney, Weller, Sutton, Bruce, and Schut (1985) have suggested that closure of the back can be safely delayed for at least 1 week after birth if antibiotic therapy is used to lessen the possibility of infection. Although the defect can be larger or smaller, most lesions are 2–4 inches in length and involve three or four vertebrae (Myers, Cerone, & Olson, 1981). The surgeon carefully preserves the neural tissue in the center of the protruding sac and excises redundant membrane. The spinal sac and lining of the spine are then closed over the neural elements, and the skin is brought across for closure. Thus, the surgery involves placement of the nervous tissue into the spinal column, attainment of a watertight closure of the dura lining, and coverage of the defect with available muscle and skin (Hammock & Milhorat, 1982).

The main consideration in surgical closure is to avoid infection. Leakage of cerebral spinal fluid from the sac may lead to infection, therefore indicating the need to close the open spine quickly. Infection of the spinal fluid can result in meningitis. In general, the operation does not improve the functional status of the spinal cord and nerves, but it may prevent complications.

In older children, other forms of neurosurgery may be indicated (Shurtleff, 1983). There may be a progressive loss of muscle function in the legs or urinary sphincters, or the child may complain of pain or tingling in either the upper or lower extremities. Surgery may be conducted to resolve problems related to pressure on the nerves due to: 1) scarring or tethering of the cord, 2) an abnormal collection of fluid in the spinal cord (hydromyelia), or 3) formation of abnormal tissue called dermoids or lipomas.

HYDROCEPHALUS AND SHUNTS

Under normal circumstances, cerebrospinal fluid circulates throughout the brain and spinal cord before being absorbed by the body. Since there is a continuous secretion of this clear fluid by three ventricles (cavities) deep within the brain, a precise amount of fluid must be absorbed by the body in order to maintain the proper amount. The absorption occurs as the cerebrospinal fluid exits through a fourth ventricle to the outer surface of the brain and spinal cord, and eventually enters the blood stream. This mechanism of production and absorption of cerebrospinal fluid ensures a stable fluid pressure.

In the majority of children with myelomeningocele, normal cerebrospinal fluid circulation is blocked (Badell-Ribera, 1985). As a result, there is excessive accumulation of the fluid in the ventricles of the brain. These cavities distend because of the trapped fluid, which causes compression on the brain tissue and enlargement of the head. This condition is termed hydrocephalus and can eventually result in brain damage and even death. The incidence of hydrocephalus associated with myelomeningocele varies according to the site of the lesion; that is, the higher the lesion, the greater the incidence.

The possible development of hydrocephalus can be monitored by routinely measuring the circumference of the child's head and comparing its size to norms of children the same age. Thus, the rate of growth of the head can be carefully followed. Another method is the use of a procedure termed a brain scan (CAT or EMI scan). This noninvasive, painless procedure takes multiple X rays of the brain. These X rays are converted by an instrument into electrical impulses, which are processed by a computer to show images on a television screen. Photographs of the images can be made. Thus, the size and shape of the brain and its ventricles can be examined. In the case of hydrocephalus, there is an increase in the size of the ventricles, with a commensurate decrease in the thickness of the brain tissue.

If it appears that hydrocephalus is developing, the neurosurgeon may perform a shunting procedure to provide drainage to the blocked ventricles. This procedure may be performed in the newborn period or any time thereafter. A flexible tube made of plastic or silicone rubber is inserted through a small opening in the skull and leads from a brain ventricle, underneath the skin of the head and neck, to drain the excess spinal fluid into either the heart (ventriculo-atrial shunt) or the abdominal cavity (ventriculoperitoneal shunt). The latter procedure is the most common. An extra length of the tubing is provided to allow for the child's physical growth. These shunt systems can have various designs, but all include a one-way valve to prevent a backward flow of the cerebrospinal fluid. Figure 4.1 diagrams the two shunting procedures.

In a child with a shunt, the tube can usually be felt under the skin behind the right ear. However, it is occasionally placed on the left side, or bilaterally if required. Although the tube and shunt valve do not require special care, it is recommended that this area be free of undue pressure. Pressing deeply onto the tube is contraindicated. A child with a shunt is not restricted from activities unless specified by a physician. The only movement that is usually to be avoided is prolonged hanging upside-down, as this position may interfere with the flow of fluid and disrupt the valvular function of the shunt.

A shunt may have to be replaced due to obstruction, malfunctioning of the valve, or growth of the child. Parents and professionals need to be able to recognize the warning signs that may indicate possible malfunction of the shunt. Safety requires that the presence of any warning signs be brought to the attention of a physician. Such warning signs include:

1. Increase in head size
2. Behavioral changes such as extreme irritability or fussiness

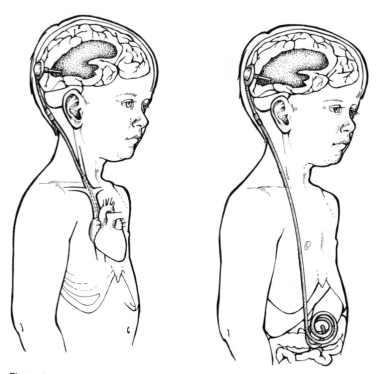

Figure 4.1. Ventriculoatrial shunt (left) and ventriculoperitoneal shunt (right).

3. Increase in sleepiness
4. Seizures
5. Diminished reaction to the environment, or lethargy
6. Forceful vomiting
7. Swelling or redness of the skin in the area of the shunt
8. Headaches
9. "Setting sun" eyes (iris only partially visible due to a downward gaze)

SPINAL DEFORMITIES

Types of Spinal Deformities

The most commonly seen spinal deformities in children with myelome-ningocele are scoliosis, kyphosis, and lordosis. A scoliosis is a lateral bend or side-to-side curvature of the spine, which may be accompanied in varying degrees by rotation of the vertebral column. When an increased kyphosis is present, a hunchback posture results in which there is an exaggeration of the normal slight posterior convexity of the thoracic spine. An increased lordosis or sway-back posture is an exaggeration of the anterior convexity of the lumbar curve. The lumbar portion of the spinal column is in extreme extension, with an anterior tilt of the pelvis and an increased arch of the lower back. An increased lordosis is frequently a compensation for hip flexion contractures, the absence of hip extensor activity, and/or the result of an increased thoracic kyphosis. A child may have one distinct type of spinal deformity or any combination of these curvatures.

Spinal deformities may be the result of congenital anomalies of the vertebral column (i.e., they may be present at birth) or may be acquired over time as a result of imbalance in trunk musculature, abnormal muscle tone, or orthopaedic complications such as a dislocated hip. Due to the my-elomeningocele, the spine may be malformed at the site of the lesion. The resulting spinal curvature may not progress significantly (that is, the degree of the curve may remain the same over time), or it may undergo a continual progression resulting in a marked deformity.

The imbalance in the trunk musculature is due to absent or insufficient nerve innervation to the muscles at and below the level of lesion. The influence of muscle imbalance on the spine is an uneven pull from the muscles attached to the vertebral column. Consequently, asymmetrical forces acting on the spine may cause a curvature. A spinal curve may also be caused by an extensive degree of muscle paralysis in which there is a lack of muscle support to the spine. In some cases, spasticity may contribute to the development of a curvature. The extent to which the presence of spasticity results in a spinal deformity depends on the degree to which it creates an uneven pull of the muscles. For example, a curvature may result when there is increased muscle tone on one side of the spine and decreased tone on the other.

A dislocated hip may contribute to a spinal deformity indirectly through the influence of positioning. If one hip is dislocated, resulting in an asymmetry of the pelvis, a compensatory scoliosis may occur. For example, a contracture of the adductor and flexor muscles of one hip can lead to a dislocation of that hip. A pelvic asymmetry may therefore be present, and the child will tend to sit on the buttock of the sound hip. To keep from falling to that side, the child laterally flexes the trunk away from the weight-bearing side. A compensatory scoliosis results, with the concavity of the curve on the side of the dislocated hip (Swinyard, 1980).

Spinal curvatures are classified according to the presence or absence of fixed deformities of the vertebral column. On the one hand, curvatures that are accompanied by actual fixed deformities of the vertebrae are referred to as structural deformities. The curve is permanent and can be observed at all times, regardless of the position of the child. Curves resulting from congenital anomalies of the spine are considered to be structural deformities.

Nonstructural or functional curves, on the other hand, are those that are flexible (not fixed) and reversible. They can be corrected through proper positioning of the child to achieve an optimal posture. For example, a child who sits asymmetrically with a compensatory scoliosis may achieve a straight spine when handled by a therapist or when seated symmetrically with proper external support. Functional curves usually result from muscle imbalance, abnormal muscle tone, or postural asymmetry due to a dislocated hip. In some circumstances, a functional curve can progress over time to a fixed, structural deformity.

Management of Spinal Deformities

Management of spinal deformities includes both nonsurgical (conservative) and surgical approaches. Physical therapy may be an adjunct to treatment with either approach.

Conservative Approaches Nonoperative orthopaedic management focuses on the use of an orthosis to prevent an increase in the curve or to decrease the curve in cases of a functional deformity. If a structural deformity is present, application of an orthosis may provide some improved alignment but generally does not correct the curvature.

A molded, plastic body jacket is the most common orthosis used with the young child. These thoraco-lumbar jackets are vests made of malleable plastic that are molded to the child's trunk to maintain symmetry of the spine. For this intervention to be effective, the jacket is usually worn by the child 23 hours a day. It is removed only for purposes of bathing and hygiene. The Milwaukee brace and various types of low-profile braces are occasionally used with the older child when an orthosis is the treatment of choice.

Surgical Approaches Surgical intervention may be indicated in more severe cases, when conservative methods have failed to prevent the progression of a curvature. The goal of surgery is to straighten the spine as much as possible through spinal instrumentation and fusion of the involved vertebrae. Active and passive range of motion of the trunk may be limited postsurgically and may result in some loss of mobility. However, this limitation is generally more acceptable than an increasing spinal deformity. Since fusion inhibits bone growth, surgical procedures are deferred whenever possible until most spinal growth has occurred, that is, until early adolescence. Occasionally surgery is required at a younger age due to the progressive nature of the deformity.

Different surgical procedures are employed for spinal fusion with or without metal supports (Brown, 1978; Hall & Poitras, 1977; Leatherman & Dickson, 1978; Piggott, 1980). The spinal column can be held firmly in place with rods, cables, or plates. In the Harrington rod procedure, a rod holds the spine in the correct position until the fusion is solidly healed. This procedure generally requires 9 months to a year of postoperative casting. Segmental instrumentation is another technique, in which the spine is wired to two L-shaped rods. The advantage of this procedure is that it does not require postoperative immobilization in a cast. However, a brace is frequently worn for a few months after surgery. This segmental instrumentation technique is used for correction of a scoliosis or kyphosis.

Therapeutic Intervention

As noted earlier, physical therapy may be a component of either a conservative or a surgical approach. The focus of therapeutic intervention is to prevent or reduce the tendency toward a spinal deformity. The goals of therapy are structured to: 1) maintain or increase the range of motion of the trunk, 2) promote symmetry of the trunk, and 3) strengthen weak musculature. If the child is capable, it is important to perform a manual muscle test in order to develop a specific exercise program to strengthen the identified weak muscles. (Testing may be difficult for preschool children who cannot follow the required verbal instructions.) It appears, however, that once the child develops a true scoliosis, a pure exercise program is not generally effective unless combined with the use of an orthotic device.

An essential aspect of intervention is the promotion of symmetry of the trunk and elongation (lengthening) of shortened trunk muscles. With the young child, these goals are promoted by maintaining alignment of the trunk and spine in all positions.

1. When lying on the back, the child's head, arms, and legs should be oriented toward the body midline. This goal can be accomplished by supporting the head and trunk with appropriately placed cushions to keep the child in a symmetrical position. Toys should be presented at the midline.
2. The side-lying position may encourage symmetrical alignment of the trunk. Pillows and cushions may be beneficial to support specific body

parts. A side-lyer may be used with the young or more physically involved child.

3. In the sitting position, there is a tendency toward trunk asymmetry due to the influence of gravity. Lateral support can be provided, to correct the functional curve or to accommodate the structural curve, in order to encourage as much symmetry as possible (see Chapter 5).

4. Braces and a corset assist symmetry of the trunk during standing. An erect, symmetrical posture is the goal.

In addition to proper positioning, symmetry and muscle elongation are also achieved during movement-oriented activities. Use of mobile surfaces such as an adult's lap, a ball, or a bolster encourages trunk elongation and develops an equal ability to weight-shift the trunk toward both sides. On a large therapy ball, for example, the young child can be facilitated to assume sitting from the prone position. It is important to practice this transitional movement equally to both sides. Chapter 3 discusses handling activities to achieve symmetry in the young child.

The use of active exercise with a child under 5 years of age is generally difficult, but is possible through the use of imaginative games. The following active exercises incorporated into play emphasize elongation of trunk musculature:

1. Touching the toes in the long-sitting position: With the legs straight out in front of the body while sitting on the floor, the child reaches with two hands to remove and replace hand or finger puppets that are placed on his or her feet or toes. A similar activity involves "painting" the lower extremities with a brush and water.

2. Rotating the upper trunk in the long-sitting position: The adult rolls a ball to alternating sides of the child. The child must twist the trunk in order to catch the ball with two hands and then roll it back to the adult. Other activities can be structured to require the child to pick up objects or toys (e.g., ring stacks, puzzles, and shape sorters) on one side and reach around to place them on the other side.

3. Rotating in diagonal patterns when seated or standing: Mobility of the trunk is encouraged by having the child perform rotational movements of the trunk in diagonal patterns. That is, the child alternates between rotation of the trunk into flexion and rotation of the trunk into extension. The child begins in a sitting or standing position that permits toys to be placed to one side at a level lower than the hips. The child reaches across the body and downward for a toy with the arm that is on the opposite side from the toy (i.e., rotation of the trunk into flexion). The child then comes up to resume an erect posture and switches the toy to the other hand. Next the child reaches across to the opposite side to place the toy on a high surface behind the body (i.e., rotation of the trunk into extension). Repetitions of this movement sequence can be incorporated into a variety

of games. The child can practice this activity in both directions, by reaching down to the left side and transferring the toy up to the right or by reaching down to the right side and transferring the toy up to the left.

Children with high lumbar lesions commonly have overactive trunk extensors and unopposed action of hip flexors that result in an increased lordotic posture when standing. Activities to strengthen the abdominal muscles are important in developing more normal pelvic control and decreasing the lordosis. The following activities emphasize abdominal function:

1. Rolling activities with rotation of the upper and lower trunk.
2. Assuming sitting from a side-lying position.
3. Activating abdominal muscles when seated on a therapy ball: With the child in a ring or in a long-sitting position on a therapy ball, the adult slightly moves the ball to facilitate a backward weight shift of the child's trunk. When the shoulders of the child are posterior in alignment to the hips (center of gravity behind the hips), the abdominal muscles are activated to maintain the sitting position. Caution is needed to ensure that the child does not compensate for weak abdominal muscles by use of the hip flexors pulling the pelvis into an anterior tilt. (In this case, the child brings the trunk forward, so that the shoulders are anterior to the line of the hips and the abdominal muscles become inactive).
4. Reaching toward the knees in the supine position.
5. Modified sit-ups: The child is semireclined on a wedge, with the legs bent at hips and knees and the feet flat on the floor. The child lifts the head (chin tuck and neck flexion) and reaches forward with both hands in order to assist the rise of the body into a sitting position.
6. Bottom-lifting games: In the supine position, the child brings the legs over the head in order to lift the buttocks off the floor. With the infant, this activity is accomplished through hand-to-feet or feet-to-mouth play.

In some cases, strengthening of the arms is indicated in the management of spinal curvature to promote more symmetrical muscle activity. Symmetrical weight-bearing activities on the upper extremities can provide this bilateral strengthening. Activities are graded by gradually increasing the degree of movement required against gravity. An example of this principle is to begin weight-bearing activities in the prone-on-elbows position, progressing to the prone-on–extended arms position, and finally to modified push-ups with the child's trunk partially supported on a wedge. The wedge helps to prevent a lordotic posture of the low back.

A follow-up activity in this same position is to have the child maintain a weight-bearing position on one extended arm while reaching out with the other arm (full shoulder flexion). Trunk muscles on the same side as the reaching arm are elongated, thus decreasing the tendency toward shortening (lateral flexion) of that side. A sequenced program of progressive resistive exercises is appropriate, as long as spasticity is not present in the arms.

Physical therapy intervention for a kyphosis emphasizes controlled trunk extension. Suggested intervention includes weight-bearing activities on straight (extended) arms in the prone-lying position, the propelling of a scooter board in the prone position, and reaching activities while in the prone-lying position over a large ball. In sitting, trunk extension is reinforced by reaching up past the height of the shoulders (over 90 degrees of shoulder flexion). In some children, a kyphosis in sitting may result from increased extensor tone in the hips. In such cases, the sitting posture is characterized by a rounded back in order to shift the body weight forward to maintain balance. Intervention begins with inhibiting excessive muscle tone prior to facilitating normal, controlled extensor movements of the trunk as described.

Physical therapy following surgery requires a very individualized program based on collaborative treatment planning with the orthopaedic surgeon. Depending on the child, intervention may focus on increasing muscle strength throughout the body when muscle tone is normal, decreasing muscle imbalance, and increasing independent mobility and functional motor skills.

HIP DISLOCATIONS

Definition and Diagnosis

The musculature surrounding the hip joint receives its nerve supply primarily from L-1 through S-1 (the first lumbar spinal nerve through the first sacral nerve). Consequently, the muscle imbalance that results from middle lumbar lesions places the hip joint at risk for dislocaton or subluxation. The hip flexors and adductors, which are innervated at L-1 and L-2, have a higher innervation level than the hip extensors and abductors (gluteus maximus and medius), which are innervated at L-4, L-5, and S-1. The child with a lesion at the L-2, L-3, and L-4 level is most at risk for a dislocation, which may be present at birth or may develop within the first few years of life. The dislocation can be unilateral or bilateral.

The hip is a ball-and-socket joint in which the spherical head of the femur (the long bone of the thigh) rests in a round socket, the acetabulum of the pelvis. When a hip is dislocated, the femoral head rests completely outside the acetabulum, although it is still within the capsule or lining of the joint. The joint capsule consists of the soft tissue structures surrounding the joint including ligaments, tendons, and connective tissue.

In a subluxation, the head of the femur is able to slip partially outside the confines of the socket because of the looseness of the joint and the laxity of its supportive structures. A subluxation can progressively worsen until the joint partially or completely dislocates. For this reason, a hip subluxation is sometimes referred to as a partial dislocation. A subluxation of the hip can usually be realigned when the hip is in a position of 90 degrees of flexion and full abduction (hips moved out away from the body midline). The procedure for manually realigning the hips is called manual reduction. If the hip is subluxed, the subluxation usually occurs when the hips are flexed and adducted.

Dislocation or subluxation results in instability of the total hip joint, and its bony development then tends to be abnormal. Consequently, early detection focuses on assessing the stability of this joint. When there is suspicion of a joint problem, X rays are necessary for a definite diagnosis by the physician. The most common methods for clinical evaluation of the hips in the newborn and infant are the Ortolani and Barlows procedures.

An Ortolani test is performed with the child placed in the supine position with both hips adducted. The examiner then abducts both lower extremities while pulling slightly anteriorly. If a hip is initially dislocated, the head of the femur will move into the acetabulum. Administering the Barlows test starts with the child in the supine position with both hips abducted. As the examiner adducts the lower extremities, the hips are pressed downward. If a hip is unstable, it will dislocate posteriorly from the joint with a resultant palpable "clunk." Therefore, the Ortolani test reduces the hip that is resting in a dislocated position, whereas the Barlows test dislocates a hip that is in the joint when that hip is positioned in abduction.

The Ortolani test is important in early detection of a hip dislocation, but it becomes progressively more difficult to elicit the described response the longer the hip remains out of the joint. Neither test is valid once the child's lower extremity stiffens or becomes tight in a dislocated position, since the hip can no longer be reduced or alternately dislodged from the joint.

Joint instability is also indicated if there is a limitation of hip abduction when passive range of motion is tested. In the normal infant and toddler, 90 degrees of hip abduction is generally achieved when the hips are flexed to 90 degrees. When the hips are dislocated, there will be limitation in the range of possible abduction. If the infant has a unilateral dislocation, a difference in the abduction range of the two hips will be apparent. Thus, it is often more difficult to detect a bilateral dislocation than a unilateral one. Other observable signs of a hip dislocation include asymmetry of skin folds on the medial aspects of the thighs and an apparent discrepancy in leg length.

Management of Hip Dislocations

If a dislocation of the hip is suspected, it should be brought to the immediate attention of the child's pediatrician and orthopaedic surgeon. There is general agreement within the medical field that early diagnosis and treatment affords the most favorable results in management of dislocated hips. Early treatment decreases further hip joint deformities and reduces the tendency toward a pelvic obliquity (asymmetry) and scoliosis, which can be common secondary complications.

Conservative Approaches Generally, conservative management in the neonatal period involves manual reduction of the hips, followed by maintenance of the hip in the stable abducted position. The orthopaedic surgeon may require this position to be maintained beyond the first year of life. Several devices and methods are used to keep the hips flexed and abducted, such as double or triple diapering, the use of a Frejka pillow splint or a Pavlik harness, and occasionally the application of a hip spica cast. By maintaining the hip in an abducted position, the lining around the joint may tighten and become secure enough to keep the hip within the joint. This approach has varying degrees of success when used in the treatment of dislocated hips in infants with myelomeningocele.

Management of hip dislocation is often complex and difficult since the initial causative factors remain unchanged. The muscular imbalance or inactivity resulting from the spinal lesion continues to influence the position of the hip. Maintenance of hip joint alignment by the methods described may not offer adequate stability at the hips for weight bearing. Therefore, surgical means of reduction may at times be necessary to promote proper alignment and stability of the hip joint.

Surgical Approaches Numerous surgical procedures are available to promote hip stabilization (Carroll, 1978; Feiwell, Sakai, & Blatt, 1978; Menelaus, 1980; Nason, 1982; Sharrard, 1983). For example, hip stability can be increased by the Sharrard procedure, or iliopsoas transfer. This operation attempts to decrease the muscular imbalance around the hip by transferring the iliopsoas, a primary hip flexor, to a lateral and more posterior position. This procedure usually eliminates the iliopsoas as a deforming force and, in many instances, increases it function as a hip abductor. An obturator neurectomy (a partial excision of the nerve supply to the hip adductors) can also be performed in order to reduce the strength of hip adduction. Muscle transfers, releases, or tenotomies, usually of hip adductors and the iliopsoas, are also common surgical procedures. At times, a varus osteotomy of the femur is employed to realign the femoral head in the acetabulum. If the configuration of the acetabulum is inadequate, it can be reshaped to form a better socket (e.g., through a Stahli "shelf" procedure or a Chiari osteotomy of the pelvis).

Riggins, Kraus, and Fontanetta (1983) have suggested that current surgical procedures to correct hip dislocations due to myelomeningocele have a limited positive influence on ambulation and function. They have noted the frequent complications associated with surgical treatment, such as femoral fractures, infections, and stiffness of the hip joint. Likewise, they have cited studies that report that dislocated hips have little or no effect on the child's ability to walk (Barden, Meyer, & Stelling, 1975; Feiwell et al., 1978;

Menelaus, 1976). Structural integrity of the hips is not required for children who use a swing-to or swing-through gait while supporting the majority of their body weight on the crutches. And pain from the dislocation is rare in these children. However, these authors have suggested that surgical treatment may be required in some cases to prevent a spinal curvature if only one hip is dislocated. Most orthopaedic surgeons now strive for symmetry of the hips and may undertake a surgical procedure if there is a unilateral dislocation. A bilateral dislocation is generally not a significant handicap for the child since gait and brace requirements are not affected.

Menelaus (1980) has emphasized that the primary focus for management of the hip is to prevent and correct deformity, particularly a flexion deformity. This problem is the most common barrier to effective ambulation. The presence of dislocated hips is a second-order concern and is surgically treated only in certain cases (e.g., a unilateral dislocation, factors related to the degree of dislocation, and the ambulatory potential of the child). Menelaus has stressed that if reduction of the hips is surgically undertaken, the operation also needs to correct the deformity and muscle imbalance.

Therapeutic Intervention

Intervention for the child with dislocated hips requires a combined team approach of the orthopaedic surgeon, physical therapist, other professionals working with the child, and the child's family. Intervention focuses on reducing the tendency toward pelvic obliquity, scoliosis, and postural deformities; the elongation of overactive muscles such as the hip flexors to avoid contractures; and the development of motor skills and a means of mobility.

Therapeutic management of limited range of motion at the hips requires special consideration. Generally accepted therapeutic techniques to increase range of motion may be contraindicated in the case of dislocated hips. Appropriate treatment techniques should be determined in consultation with the orthopaedic surgeon.

Maintenance of the hips in a position of reduction through external devices provides stability to the joints but often interferes with the progression in motor development. For example, when the hips are positioned in abduction and flexion, rolling is difficult. As a consequence, various components of movement, which under normal circumstances are developed as the child practices rolling, are limited. The position of reduction may also result in a lack of pelvic mobility. Typically, at 4 months of age the normal infant begins to develop pelvic movements forward, backward, and laterally. Lack of pelvic mobility is due to the degree of hip flexion and absence of hip extension, which cause the child to remain in an anterior pelvic tilt. In such cases, the achievement of abdominal muscle control is important in order to attain a more neutral position of the pelvis.

A major goal of intervention with the young child is to provide sensory and motor experiences while the hips are maintained in the position of reduction (that is, flexion and abduction). Developmentally appropriate activities are encouraged in as normal a manner as possible in the supine, prone, and side-lying positions, thus minimizing the impact of the hip dislocation on general development.

1. In the supine position, the infant is facilitated to engage in midline-oriented play such as bringing hands to feet and bottom-lifting activities.
2. To provide prone activities, the lower extremity position is accommodated by working with the child on the adult's lap or by allowing the child's legs to remain over the edge of therapy equipment such as a bolster, ball, or mat table. Weight-bearing and weight-shifting activities on elbows and on extended arms are particularly important, since the infant may have difficulty achieving these skills independently with the hips in a reduced position.
3. Side-lying activities require similar adaptive positioning. Tasks are performed on an adult's lap or on a piece of equipment that supports the child's trunk while the legs rest off the surface and are supported by the adult. In addition to midline play, the position serves as a transitional step to encourage rolling. Rolling is facilitated from the supine to side-lying position and back, before progressing to a complete roll onto the abdomen.

A second major goal of intervention is to assist the child to develop functional mobility skills in order to explore the environment. Intervention emphasizes movements of the trunk and upper extremities. However, the lower limbs should not be excluded in these activities, even though full movement may be restricted by the hip position if held in reduction. It may be necessary for the child to rely on upper body movement to compensate for limitations in the legs.

Propulsion backward, and later forward, in the prone position can be assisted by having the child progress down an inclined surface such as a wedge. A scooter board can also be used in the prone-lying position. The child will favor ring sitting if in the position of reduction. Scooting on the buttocks is possible once the child has developed security in this sitting position. Usually, bottom scooting develops in a backward direction before forward and sideward mobility are achieved. The child's clothing should be adequate to afford protection against abrasion of the buttocks.

The child with dislocated hips may have initial difficulty maintaining a quadruped position and crawling, because of instability at the hips and an inability to shift weight from one side to the other. Lack of hip extension also limits crawling. Generally, children with these characteristics learn to compensate by crawling in the manner described in Chapter 3.

It is important that the therapist work closely with the orthopaedic surgeon in planning the progression to kneeling, standing, and walking when dislocation of the hips is present. These activities should be performed only when the joints of the lower extremities are in proper alignment through external control by the therapist or through an assistive device. Frequently, bilateral long-leg braces that support the legs in a neutral position are necessary for full weight bearing on the lower limbs. Even with bracing, postural deviations may be present to some degree because of the hip instability, as is the case in a lordosis and hip flexion.

DEFORMITIES OF THE KNEES

Long-leg braces are often required to support the knees because of a lack of knee extension (nonfunctional quadriceps) or to prevent medio-lateral laxity of the knee joint. The latter condition can occur due to inadequate or improper muscle forces on the knee joint. Contractures at the knee may develop in some children. If the level of lesion allows for more active quadriceps activity than opposing hamstring control, the child may have a tendency to an extension contracture at the knee. A flexion contracture of the knee may occur in a child who maintains a sitting position in a wheelchair over an extended period of time or in a child with overactive hamstrings.

Internal tibial rotation can occur when the medial hamstrings (semi-tendinosus and semimembranosus) are active and not counterbalanced by the lateral hamstring (biceps femoris). As a result, an internal tibial rotation places the lower leg out of alignment with the upper leg. Sometimes the intrauterine position can result in a true twisting of the tibia. This condition is termed internal tibial torsion and may be perpetuated by the child sleeping in a tucked or flexed position at night. In other cases, an external torsion is present, possibly related to a contracture of the ilio-tibial band and malalignment of the bones (talus and navicular) in the equinovarus foot (Madden & Bchir, 1977). If either condition is persistent or severe, a derotation osteotomy of the tibia can be performed to correct the problem. Most commonly, orthopaedic surgeons recommend the use of a Denis Browne splint at night to resolve the problem in a child less than 3–4 years of age. This orthosis is composed of two shoes attached to a connecting bar. The length of the bar and the adjusted position of the shoes are specifically prescribed for the individual child.

DEFORMITIES OF THE ANKLES AND FEET

Proper positioning of the foot evenly on the floor (plantigrade position) frequently requires bracing. Typically, there is an absence or imbalance of muscle action at the ankle and foot. In addition, the foot is usually anesthetic (without feeling) and prone to pressure sores. Due to dysfunction of the gastrocnemius and soleus muscles, the brace must prevent dorsiflexion past 90 degrees to attain stability of the ankle. This can be achieved by using a plastic posterior shell orthosis that has a rigid ankle, or a double upright metal brace with an anterior stop mechanism. Plastic, total contact bracing has emerged as a preferred method of bracing for children with spina bifida.

A wide variety of ankle and foot deformities occur in children with myelomeningocele. A *calcaneovalgus deformity* (see Figure 4.2) may occur as a result of strong activity of the anterior tibial muscles and absence of the gastrocnemius and soleus muscles. The foot is pulled up and outward in a dorsiflexed posture. Consequently, pressure is placed on the heel and not on the sole of the foot. Soft tissue transfer of the anterior tibial tendon may be required to achieve a plantigrade foot, or the tendon may be released to eliminate its deforming force. In contrast, an *equinovarus deformity* (see Figure 4.3) is one in which the foot is pointed down and both the forefoot and hindfoot are in a varus or medially deviated position. An equinovarus deformity occurs frequently as an associated congenital anomaly in children with myelomeningocele. Many times casting may correct the deformity, although care must be taken in casting a child with an anesthetic foot. In more severe cases, surgical soft tissue releases may be necessary to achieve an optimal position of the foot.

A *vertical talus deformity* (rigid rocker bottom foot) (see Figure 4.4) is another common congenital anomaly. Surgical intervention is usually required since this defect can rarely be corrected by casting. In a *varus deformity,* the forefoot or hindfoot is in an inverted position. This abnormality may be resolved by either a lateral transfer of the involved muscles or, more commonly, by releasing the offending tendons to allow the foot to be placed in a neutral position.

In some children, the fibula of the lower leg grows at a slower pace than the adjacent tibia because of inactivity of the peroneal and other muscles attached to the fibula (Nason, 1982). This condition results in a *valgus tilt* at the ankle joint. That is, the ankle turns out, producing a pronation deformity of the foot. Other problems occasionally noted include *flexion contractures and clawing of the toes*. The latter condition is brought about by extrinsic muscles acting in the absence of intrinsic muscle action. This phenomenon may be seen in children with sacral lesions.

In summary, deformities of the feet in children with myelomeningocele vary markedly and are due to a wide variety of causes. The problem may be related to such factors as abnormal positioning *in utero,* imbalanced muscle pull, and/or a true bony deformity. Furthermore, completely different deformities can occur in the separate feet of one child. This discrepancy may be related to the previously mentioned factors or due to differing degrees of innervation to the muscles of each lower extremity.

The child who exhibits congenital foot deformities is followed closely by an orthopaedic surgeon. The physician determines the severity of the ankle anomaly and chooses the type of intervention. The treatment may include one or more of the following: passive range of motion exercises to the talocalcaneal

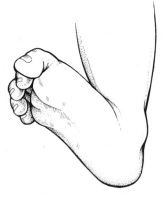

Figure 4.2. A common foot deformity: calcaneovalgus.

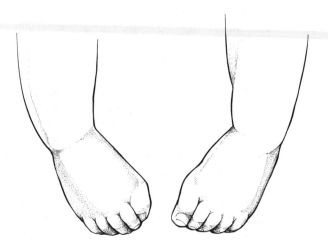

Figure 4.3. A common foot deformity: equinovarus.

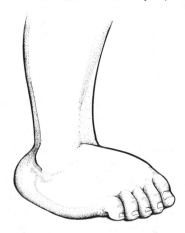

Figure 4.4. A common foot deformity: vertical talus.

and subtalar (ankle) joints, short-leg casts, plastic ankle/foot orthoses (with anterior shell if indicated), and corrective surgery.

The physician frequently begins by recommending passive range of motion exercises. If daily ranging exercises are not sufficient to maintain neutral ankle alignment, casts or orthoses are often applied. Surgery is indicated when all conservative means of intervention have proven inadequate. Following surgery, the physician usually casts the child's lower extremities below the knee to maintain the corrected ankle alignment. When the casts are removed, orthoses are applied immediately to prevent any future deformity from occurring.

The therapist's role during this period is to continue working on the goals that were set initially for the child and that are not influenced by the child's decreased ankle mobility. These goals would probably include increasing the functional strength or power of the upper extremities and the trunk as well as providing a means of independent mobility, which may require the use of a wheelchair or scooter board during the time that the child is nonambulatory. Once the casts are removed postoperatively, therapy includes a training progression toward ambulation. Determination of the child's weight-bearing status and use of orthotic devices is routinely decided by the attending physician.

OSTEOPOROSIS

Active muscular pull and weight bearing have been shown to promote bone growth. A loss of bone substance due to inactivity and lack of weight bearing is called disuse osteoporosis. Children with myelomeningocele are predisposed to osteoporosis as a result of motor involvement. Immobility and limited activity level disturb the normal calcium metabolism required for bone growth. As a result, bones may become thin and porous and be susceptible to fractures.

The highest incidence of spontaneous leg fractures in children with myelomeningocele occurs during the preschool years (Rickard, Brady, & Gresham, 1977). Most commonly, the fracture is sustained after the leg has been immobilized in a cast after surgery or following treatment of another fracture. The cause of the fracture is typically minor, such as a rough transfer or merely rolling over in bed. Since the child may be unaware of the injury, adults need to be alert to the signs of inflammation that result from trauma, including redness, swelling, and warmth.

Prevention of osteoporosis and its complications entails proper nutritional management and the promotion of weight bearing particularly in standing. Supported upright positioning can be achieved using a prone stander, parapodium, tilt table, and/or braces. Most orthopaedic surgeons agree that it is important to get children upright in their early years regardless of their level of neurological involvement. The effect of weight bearing is critical for proper mineralization and development of bony structures of the lower extremities.

SKIN CARE

The total or partial loss of sensation (touch, pain, and temperature) deprives the young child of protective mechanisms against trauma. Care must be taken to prevent injury to anesthetic areas at and below the level of lesion. Pressure and friction can irritate the skin, causing it to be reddened, warm, or blistered. When sensation is partially intact, the skin may also feel tender. If the skin is broken, the sore is commonly referred to as a decubitus ulcer, pressure sore, bedsore, or skin ulcer. Adherence to the following safety precautions is recommended when there is a loss of sensation:

1. Contact of the skin with uneven, rough or sharp surfaces should be avoided. Even creases in chair seats, clothing, or bedding can cause pressure sores.
2. Gentle handling of the legs during transfers and daily care should be encouraged.
3. Tight-fitting clothes and shoes should be avoided.
4. Extremes in temperature of such surfaces as hot and cold water pipes, radiators, and car seats exposed to the sun can be dangerous. In severe winter climates, prolonged exposure to the cold places the child at risk for frostbite, especially of the feet and toes.
5. Clothing should be worn most of the time, particularly if the child is independently mobile in the environment. Long pants with extra padding sewn at the knees are helpful for the child who is an active crawler. Shoes and socks are essential to protect feet that lack sensation. On the beach, sneakers and socks are frequently recommended to prevent foot injury.
6. The carrying of pencils, toys, and other items in the pockets of pants or in the wheelchair should be discouraged. Inadvertent sitting on them can injure the skin. Carrying bags are commercially available that attach to the back of the wheelchair for storing personal items, or side pouches can be secured to the armrests for more convenient access to a storage area.
7. Special back and seat cushions for the wheelchair may prevent pressure sores from developing. A child with a marked kyphosis may require a customized back cushion for proper protection.

Children may lack awareness of injury to the skin after it has occurred. The adult needs to teach the young child as early as possible to inspect anesthetic skin on a regular daily basis. This practice reinforces the child's awareness of possible injury and results in early detection of reddened areas that may lead to pressure sores. The following guidelines promote the maintenance of healthy skin:

1. Wet and soiled diapers should be changed as soon as possible.
2. Areas of prolonged redness or blistering should be brought to the attention of a nurse or physician. Proper and timely care will prevent infection.

3. The skin should be thoroughly checked for reddened pressure areas after removal of braces, splints, and shoes.
4. Prolonged static sitting by the nonambulatory child may result in pressure sores. Positioning should be changed by the child or caregiver at least every 1–2 hours. Readjustment of the sitting posture to redistribute weight and pressure should occur more frequently. A child in a wheelchair can push the palms against the armrests to lift the body up. The child should be encouraged to perform these "push-ups" on a routine basis to relieve pressure on the buttocks.

The major mode of treatment for a decubitus ulcer is to remove pressure from the injured area. A child may be required to stay in a semiprone or prone position if the pressure sore is on the back or buttocks. Children with spina bifida are especially susceptible to ulcerations of the lower extremities and may need to discontinue wearing orthoses and/or shoes until healing of the area is attained. The skin should be exposed to the air as much as possible; 20- to 30-minute periods of exposure at least three or four times a day are usually recommended. Close medical attention is needed to ensure optimal recovery.

Children with myelomeningocele may have reduced circulation due to paralysis and muscle weakness. Normally, muscles act as a pump to aid the circulation of blood throughout the body. Loss of this muscular pumping action predisposes the child to lowered superficial skin temperature. For example, legs and feet are often cold to the touch and may appear discolored or bluish. The tendency toward decreased circulation is reduced by avoiding extreme changes in temperature and dressing appropriately in cold weather. The diminished circulation also affects the skin's healing process. Cuts and scrapes may take longer to heal, and swelling may be unusually prolonged at an injured area. When swelling is present, elevation of the area is recommended to decrease the pooling of fluid, which results from impaired circulation.

◇ CHAPTER 5 ◇

Positioning
and Mobility

GUIDELINES FOR A PROPER SITTING POSTURE AND ALTERNATIVE POSITIONS appropriate to the home and classroom are discussed in this chapter. Wheelchairs are then addressed, regarding appropriate fit, basic management, and techniques for maneuvering in a variety of circumstances. The different types of braces that can help to achieve standing and ambulation are then reviewed, as are other mobility aids.

POSITIONING

Proper positioning at home and in the classroom is important for many reasons: to discourage the development of orthopaedic deformities (e.g., joint contractures, spinal deformities), to avoid accidents, to maintain good skin care, to achieve functional use of the upper extremities, and to facilitate optimal learning and independence. It is important for the child to have a good posture in sitting as well as alternative positions that can be assumed in the course of the day.

Proper Sitting Posture

General principles need to be kept in mind in order to achieve a good sitting posture in a regular chair. The child should have the hips well back into the chair, sitting equally on both buttocks. With the pelvis properly placed, the trunk is usually in erect alignment and the legs are positioned to provide an adequate base of support for sitting. A right angle (90 degrees of flexion) is maintained at the hip, knee, and ankle joints.

The size of the chair is critical in order for proper positioning to occur. The height of the chair is important to avoid dangling feet. The feet should rest firmly on the floor or on a footrest. In addition, the depth of the chair seat should provide full support from the buttocks to an inch or so behind the knees. The child's body weight is thus distributed on the buttocks and length of the thighs for a comfortable sitting base. If the seat of the chair is too short, balance and sitting tolerance will be poor. If the seat is too long, the child will tend to slump in the chair in a semireclining fashion or try to accommodate by sitting on the front edge of the seat without back support. Both of these postures undermine the child's ability to engage in activities with postural security.

Some modifications of a regular chair or wheelchair may be required for children with marked muscle weakness or an imbalance of muscle use in the trunk. These children may tend to sit asymmetrically on one buttock and/or list the trunk laterally to the side. Maintaining symmetrical hip and trunk alignment while seated may help prevent the development of a scoliosis (curvature of the spine). The pelvis can be held in proper alignment by the use of hip control guides which keep the pelvis from deviating in an undesired direction. Lateral supports can be attached to the chair to prevent the trunk from leaning toward one side. If the child is in a wheelchair or enclosed seat, rolled towels may provide temporary support to the sides of the trunk or legs to achieve symmetry.

These suggestions for adaptive positioning may or may not be required if the child has an orthosis (braces, pelvic band, and/or corset). Although braces keep the child's joints in alignment, there is still some degree of movement within the braces. It is not unusual to see a totally braced child sitting asymmetrically. Regardless of the level of function, safety is always a priority. Therefore, a seatbelt is indicated when there is poor postural control. In general, a seatbelt should progress from the base of the chair across the hips at a 45-degree angle and attach above the groin. This line of pull keeps the hips well back in the chair and assists desired alignment of the pelvis, which is the key point of control for sitting. A seatbelt wrapped around the waist is uncomfortable, impairs breathing patterns, and fails to provide the proper support. The child will tend to slide under the seatbelt into a semireclining position.

The height of the table also warrants attention. When seated in a chair, the child should be able to rest the elbows comfortably on the table surface, slightly toward the side. This distance of the work surface from the child facilitates visual-motor skills. If the table is too low, the child will collapse down toward it in a slumped posture. If the table is too high, the child will "hang" on the table with the elbows pointed out to the sides (that is, in a position of marked shoulder abduction). Commercial furniture vendors usually suggest 10-inch chairs and 20-inch tables for preschool children, but this table height is inappropriately high for most children. Instead, it is recommended that a 17- to 19-inch table be used with a sturdy wooden 10-inch chair.

Some children may require adaptation of the table surface. A child with very poor sitting balance and possibly braced to the chest may profit from a higher table height. A table approaching the child's nipple level may assist the maintenance of an erect trunk and provide more support for propping on the elbows. Other children have the best posture and functional use of the arms when the work surface is inclined toward them. An inclined table surface can be achieved by placing a hard foam rubber wedge on the table or hinging a plywood board on the table that can be raised to varying heights to adjust the degree of incline. Bergen and Colangelo (1985) have described the construction of a small table easel and an easel lapboard for a wheelchair. Of course, all work surfaces must have a nonglare finish.

Alternative Positions

Young children do not maintain a static posture for a long period of time. They frequently and automatically shift their body weight and attain new positions. For children with motor handicaps who do not have this adaptive control, it is essential to provide a variety of positions appropriate to the task at hand. Prolonged sitting in a chair, wheelchair, or corner of a couch at home limits the opportunity for experiential learning. It can also contribute to pressure sores, joint contractures, and even hip dislocations.

Positioning equipment can be constructed for the child or can be purchased commercially. Bergen and Colangelo (1985) and Finnie (1975) have provided guidelines for the construction of numerous positioning devices. (Appendix B lists sources for commercially available equipment.) Factors to consider in the use of adaptive positioning include:

1. Motor abilities of the child
2. Size of the home or classroom
3. Amount of storage space
4. Cost of the equipment
5. Versatility of the positioning aids

Chapter 3 discusses in detail the positioning of children to foster specific motor and functional skills. This section highlights alternative positions appropriate to the home or classroom for toddlers and preschool children. These include supine, side-lying, prone, floor-sitting, short-sitting, and standing positions.

Supine Position In general, the supine position is not beneficial for the toddler and preschool child. In this position, the child faces the ceiling, making it difficult to play with toys and to interact socially with peers. During hospitalization, the child may be placed automatically on the back for extended periods of time whether this is indicated or not.

The supine posture may be appropriate, however, for the severely involved child with marked hydrocephalus and poor control of the head and trunk. In this case, the child can lie on a wedge, with the degree of incline determined by the amount of head support required. The higher the incline, the more difficult it is to maintain the head in midline. Lateral supports can be attached to the wedge with Velcro to maintain the trunk in straight alignment. A pillow can be placed under the head to achieve a position of slight flexion. At times, a small roll may be provided under the legs to maintain flexion at the hips and knees. These adaptations inhibit the tendency toward extensor posturing of the body and facilitate the development of flexor control. Positioning the head in midline is important to inhibit the abnormal tonic neck reflexes that are commonly observed in the child with severe neurological impairment.

Side-Lying Position The side-lying position is indicated for the multiply handicapped child with limited postural control. Side lying facilitates a midline orientation, with the two hands together for swiping at objects. The posture discourages the likelihood of eliciting pathological brain stem reflexes (i.e., the tonic labyrinthine reflex and the asymmetrical tonic neck reflex). If supported in side lying, the child can engage in activities with minimal postural demands. If the child actively maintains the position, however, it encourages the development of extensor and flexor muscles working together to provide controlled lateral movement.

When positioning a child in side lying on the floor or wedge, the head should be resting on a pillow in slight flexion, which allows for proper alignment in the midline. Otherwise, the head tends to "hang" laterally toward the floor. Depending on individual needs, the lower extremities are positioned in different ways. Commonly, the legs are in bilateral hip and knee flexion or positioned with the weight-bearing leg in extension and the upper, non–weight-bearing leg in hip and knee flexion. In this posture, extension at the hip fosters elongation (or lengthening) of the trunk on the weight-bearing side. When a child is in side lying, the adult presents toys and educational materials in an appropriate visual orientation that accommodates for the horizontal position of the child. Care is also required to place the materials below the child's eye level to facilitate neck flexion and discourage head hyperextension.

Prone Position Most children with spina bifida can assume a prone-on-elbows position independently. This posture can strengthen extension of the head and trunk while developing the counterbalanced flexor control of weight bearing on the upper extremities. When reaching with one arm in play, the child experiences a weight shift and lateral flexion of the trunk. The prone position also provides an opportunity to lengthen (therapeutically stretch) tight hip flexors in order to prevent the occurrence of hip flexion contractures.

A wedge can be utilized for supported prone lying to make it easier for the child to use the arms during activity. The wedge lifts the upper trunk to facilitate spinal extension and assists in maintaining weight bearing on the arms. The height and incline of the wedge should be appropriate to the size of the child, the child's level of motor control, and the need to support body weight on the elbows or extended arms. Educational materials should be placed on the floor to encourage alignment of the head and neck with the trunk (i.e., cervical extension and flexion or "chin tuck" at the atlanto-occipital joint). Otherwise, the child will hyperextend the head and neck in order to view the activities in the classroom. Likewise, practitioners should avoid standing above the child since this will facilitate hyperextension.

Two modifications may be required to ensure desired positioning of the lower extremities. If the hips assume marked flexion, abduction, and external rotation (a froglike posture), hip guides (attached by Velcro to the wedge) can keep the legs in adduction and neutral alignment. If there is excessive plantar flexion (pointing down) of the feet, a small roll placed under the ankles will allow dorsiflexion.

A bolster can be used instead of a wedge to serve the same function. However, the bolster does not provide support to the lower torso, so there is a tendency to assume a lordotic posture. Care is necessary to ensure that the bolster is not too large in diameter, thus encouraging this "sway-back" posture of the lower trunk. The bolster can also be used for a supported quadruped position during group activities in the classroom. If the bolster is under the upper trunk in the all-fours position, it decreases the requirements of the arms to maintain weight bearing. If the bolster is close to the hips, it primarily assists the legs in supporting the body's weight.

Floor-Sitting Position   In toddler and preschool programs, many of the group and free play activities are conducted on the floor. Therefore, it is important that every child with myelomeningocele have a number of floor-sitting positions that allow for independent functioning. In general, postures that are symmetrical and provide a wide base of support are easiest to maintain, such as ring (bow) sitting or cross-legged (tailor) sitting. A child in long-leg braces with a pelvic band can assume only a long-sitting position on the floor (i.e., flexed at the hips and the legs straight out in front). If necessary, external support can be provided by placing the child against a wall or corner of the classroom, in a floor seat, or in a cutout plastic laundry basket. In this fashion, support is offered to the trunk, which frees the arms from propping to engage in activity.

For most children with spina bifida, the "W" sitting position (sitting on the buttocks between heels of the feet) is contraindicated, since it places undue stress on the hip joints in adduction and internal rotation. Side sitting is the most developmentally sophisticated floor-sitting position. It requires the child to sit asymmetrically on one buttock and to use righting reactions of lateral flexion and rotation in the trunk to maintain the posture. To be introduced to side sitting for short periods of time, the child can prop one elbow on a wooden box or low table to achieve proximal stability. The other hand is then available for manipulative play. Care must be taken that floor-sitting positions do not reinforce contractures and deformities in the lower extremities.

Short-Sitting Position   Various pieces of equipment can be used to help the child maintain a short-sitting position (i.e., right-angled sitting). Often the only required modification is a standard chair with armrests, which furnishes lateral support for postural security and safety. A commercially available bolster seat enables the child to sit in a straddle position over a stable roll. If an adult is working with the child, the preschooler can sit sideways on a regular bolster. In this short-sitting position, the child has a slightly movable surface in an anterior/posterior plane to elicit balance responses of the pelvis and trunk (that is, movements of flexion and extension). As the child reaches forward, there is a weight shift over the feet that provides a desirable weight-bearing experience.

Standing Position   There are several assistive devices to maintain a child in standing. The use of such equipment is determined by the physician and therapist on the basis of the child's medical and orthopaedic status. The most common items include a standing brace, parapodium, prone stander, standing table, and long-leg braces with a pelvic band and possibly a corset. (The standing brace and parapodium are discussed in a later section of this chapter.)

Prone standers provide an early weight-bearing experience with the trunk and legs in supported, symmetrical alignment. Weight bearing in an upright posture assists bone growth and circulation. The angle of incline of most prone standers can be varied to grade the degree of weight bearing by the lower extremities. The more erect the posture, the greater the amount of body weight supported through the legs. The child can be placed in this semistanding position, in or out of braces, to increase standing tolerance and balance. Prone standers can be purchased commercially or fabricated in various designs (Bergen & Colangelo, 1985; Finnie, 1975). They can rest against a table or maintain a free-standing position. Modifications include lateral trunk supports, adjustable footplates, and adaptations for proper placement of the legs.

A standing table may be employed by a nonambulatory child who is adequately braced. It provides a work surface enclosed within a boxlike structure that maintains the child in a safe standing position. There are limitations, however, in the use of a standing table. Frequently, the child stands asymmetrically despite the bracing. Also, since the child is enclosed in the standing box, it tends to offer a passive, overly secure position. For many children in long-leg braces, standing at a regular table is preferred. The child then has an opportunity to practice active postural control and to interact directly with peers.

WHEELCHAIRS

Whether a child is completely unable to walk or can walk using braces and crutches, a wheelchair can be of great assistance to mobility. A wheelchair has an advantage over a stroller, since it enables the child to progress from place to place without help. In cases in which independent wheelchair mobility is not feasible, a sturdy stroller that provides a firm back and seat can be used. The lightweight collapsible strollers made of nylon webbing do not offer sufficient postural stability for most young children. The toddler or preschooler tends to assume a passive, semireclining position. Measuring a child for a proper stroller is similar to the procedure employed in determining the dimensions of a wheelchair. To ensure an appropriate fit, a seat insert for the stroller can be constructed or commercially purchased.

Wheelchair independence means not only the ability to move around obstacles safely but also the ability to get in and out of the wheelchair without assistance. For this reason, it is useful for the child, parent, and practitioner to understand the construction and dynamics of the wheelchair. Figure 5.1 illustrates its major parts. In order for the child to benefit maximally, a proper fit is necessary. A chair that is too big does not provide adequate support and can hinder the child in attempting to propel the chair independently. A chair that is too small confines postural adjustments within the chair, interferes with transfers, and may cause pressure areas to develop on the skin. A commercially ordered or individually constructed seat insert may be placed in the wheelchair to provide a firm seat and back. To ensure a desirable fit, the wheelchair should be prescribed by a physician, with recommendations by the child's physical or occupational therapist. If an insert is used in a stroller or wheelchair, it must be

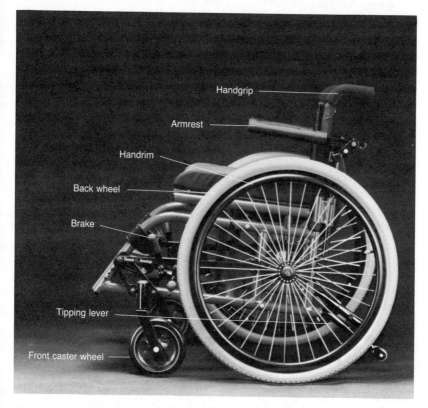

Figure 5.1. Components of a wheelchair (photo courtesy of Everest & Jennings).

firmly secured to the frame. The purpose of a seatbelt is to hold the child, not the insert.

Wheelchair Checkout

Seat Depth   If the seat is too short, the child's weight is not distributed properly along the buttocks and thighs. Therefore, excessive pressure is placed on the buttocks. If the seat is too long, the edge presses into the back of the knees causing skin irritation and decreased circulation.

The seat depth is correct when two fingers can be placed between the front of the seat and the back of the child's knees (that is, a distance of 1–2 inches).

Seat Width   If the seat is too narrow, it is difficult for the child to get in and out of the chair. Pressure areas at the sides of the legs may also develop. If the seat is too wide, there is insufficient postural support, and the child may find it difficult to propel the chair.

The seat width is correct when an adult's hand can be placed vertically between the child's hips and the sides of the chair.

Footrest Height in Relation to the Seat   If the distance between the footrests and the seat is too large, the child's legs are not adequately supported. There will be too much pressure on the thighs just above the knees since the feet are essentially dangling. If the distance between the footrests and the seat is too short, the child sits with too much hip flexion, the thighs are not supported, and the primary body weight is placed on the buttocks.

The footrests and the seat are the correct distance apart when the child's weight is supported along the major length of the thighs, the feet rest securely on the footrests, and the hips, knees, and ankles are maintained at 90 degrees of flexion.

Armrest Height   The armrests are too high if the child's shoulders are raised, as if shrugging, when the upper extremities are on the armrests. The armrests are too short if the child must lean forward to reach them.

The height is correct when the child can sit erect with the arms resting comfortably on the armrests.

Back Height   The back height should correspond to the amount of support the child needs, based on the degree of disability. In general, the back support should rise to just below the scapulae.

Basic Rules for Handling the Wheelchair

1. The seatbelt should be snug at the child's hips and worn at most times.
2. In general, a seat insert should be used to provide a firm base and back when the child is in the wheelchair.
3. When pushing a child in a wheelchair, normal strides should be taken. It is important for the adult to look ahead a minimum of 5–10 feet beyond the wheelchair so as to avoid any marked unevenness in the surface (such as a

large crack in the sidewalk) or any obstacle that might block the forward motion of the small front wheels and bring the wheelchair to a jarring halt.

4. Stopping on a graded incline should be avoided because the wheelchair could start to roll accidentally.

5. On uneven ground, it may become necessary for the adult to tip the chair onto its back wheels by stepping down onto the tipping lever. The chair is then pushed tipped backward on the rear wheels.

6. It may be easier over rough terrain for the adult to turn the chair around and pull it, rather than push it.

7. The brakes on *both* wheels should be locked whenever the chair is stationary.

8. When assisting the child to transfer out of the wheelchair, the adult should lock the brakes and move the footplates out of the way by pushing them up (in the case of stationary footrests) or by swinging them to the side (in the case of swingaway footrests). The child should not be allowed to stand on the footplates when transferring, as this practice may cause the wheelchair to tip forward.

9. If space is limited, the wheelchair can be folded when it is not in use. Most chairs can be folded by first removing any seat inserts, folding up the footrests, and then pulling up on the soft seat. Some seats have handles on them for this purpose. To open a folded chair, the adult pushes down on the lateral seat rails.

Special Techniques for Maneuvering the Wheelchair

Tilting the Wheelchair   Maneuvering the wheelchair up and down curbs and ramps may require that the chair be tilted onto its back wheels. A properly constructed chair will reach a balance point that is easy to maintain when tilted back approximately 30 degrees. To tilt the chair, the adult places one foot on the tipping lever and pushes down while simultaneously pulling back on the handgrips. When the balance point has been reached, the chair will be easy to maintain in the tilted position. The adult should not tilt the chair beyond this point as it will then become difficult to keep it from falling backward.

To return the chair to an upright position, the adult simply places one foot on the tipping lever and allows the chair to lower slowly by controlling simultaneously with the foot and hands. The chair should not be allowed to drop abruptly.

Ascending a Curb   When mounting a curb, the adult presses one foot on the tipping lever, raising the front wheels. The adult pushes the wheelchair until the front wheels are suspended over the sidewalk and the back wheels touch the curb. Then the adult lowers the front wheels onto the sidewalk and slowly lifts and rolls the back wheels up over the curb edge.

Descending a Curb   The preferred method when descending a curb is for the adult to turn the chair around so that it comes down the curb backward.

The rear wheels must be perpendicular to the edge of the curb. In order to gain stability, the adult should brace the thigh against the backrest and slowly roll the rear wheels down over the curb. Once the rear wheels are on street level, the adult pushes down on the tipping lever to raise the front wheels, and then pulls the wheelchair away from the curb. When the front wheels are clear of the curb, the tipping lever is used to lower the front wheels. The front of the chair should be a safe distance from the curb before lowering.

An alternate method for descending a curb is for the adult to align the chair facing the curb. The tipping lever is used to tilt the chair backward onto the rear wheels. The adult slowly rolls the chair forward and lets it ride down over the curb on the rear wheels. When on street level, the tipping lever and handgrips are used to lower the front wheels.

This frontal approach is less desirable than a backward descent because: 1) there is a greater likelihood of the child falling out of the chair, 2) it is more difficult to control the safe descent of the chair, and 3) it can place undue stress on the adult's back, which could cause injury. If this method is employed, the adult should take care to bend his or her legs as the chair is lowered over the curb, to prevent back strain.

Ascending a Ramp   When ascending a ramp, the wheelchair should always be pushed ahead of the adult. When age appropriate, the child can assist by pushing the handrims attached to the rear wheels. If a short rest is needed by the adult, a foot is placed under one of the rear wheels. Then the handbrakes are locked to prevent the chair from sliding backward.

Descending a Ramp   To descend a ramp, the wheelchair is turned around so the child faces uphill, and the adult brings the chair down the ramp backward. This practice has the adult positioned behind the chair so as not to lose control. If capable, the child can help control the speed of descent by putting some pressure on the handrims.

Doorways   When a child cannot assist in entering or exiting through a door, the adult should use his or her arm or leg to brace the door and at the same time pull the wheelchair through. It does not matter which way the door opens as long as one can secure it so that the door does not strike the chair when it closes.

Ascending a Short Flight of Steps   If possible, two adults should assist when ascending stairs. The wheelchair is pulled up the steps backward. One person tilts the chair back using the tipping lever and then rolls the chair up one step at a time by pulling on the handgrips. The other person holds the frame of the wheelchair in front to provide stability and balance while lifting and rolling the chair over the steps.

Descending a Short Flight of Steps   Preferably two adults should assist in lowering the chair down steps, although one person can accomplish the task safely. Probably the easiest method is to descend the stairs with the wheelchair facing forward. One adult uses the tipping lever to tilt the chair back onto the rear wheels so that the child is leaning backward and not able to fall out of the wheelchair. The other adult can stand on a lower step in front of the chair to secure the frame. The pull of gravity is the major force causing the chair to roll down each step consecutively. The adult behind the chair provides the controlling counterforce on the handgrips to keep the chair tilted at a backward angle and prevents the occurrence of a harsh bumping action at each step.

Riding Elevators When entering an elevator, the wheelchair should be brought in backward. The child and adult can then read the floor markings and are ready to exit quickly. If the child can propel the chair, the adult holds the door open. On occasion, the elevator does not stop at an even plane with the floor. It is then difficult to push the small front wheels (casters) over the unlevel surface. Assuming there is room to turn the chair around, it is easier in this situation to roll the chair out backward leading with the large rear wheels.

Electric Wheelchairs

The use of electric wheelchairs is not common in the case of young children with spina bifida. A motorized wheelchair may be helpful, however, if the child is severely disabled and has insufficient strength and control of the arms to maneuver a regular wheelchair. Since electric wheelchairs are very heavy, it is not possible to tilt them onto their rear wheels. Therefore, one must use a ramp instead of a curb. Although an electric wheelchair can safely ascend most ramps, be aware that it is not equipped with brakes. If the motor stops as the chair is ascending, the chair will begin to roll back down the incline. On a steep grade, an adult should walk behind the wheelchair as a safety precaution.

When descending a ramp in an electric wheelchair, the child faces forward. To prevent the chair from gaining undue speed, the chair can be driven in a zigzag manner down the ramp.

BRACES

The Use of Braces

Bracing plays an important role in the treatment of children with myelomeningocele. Braces (orthoses) provide support and alignment to the body for a proper posture in sitting and standing. By supporting the child who might not otherwise be able to stand, braces allow for the physiological benefits derived from being in the upright position (i.e., improved bone growth and calcification, better bladder and respiratory functions). Braces also protect the child from injury by supporting fragile bones that may easily fracture and unstable joints that may move out of alignment.

Bracing is prescribed by a physician on an individual basis, depending on the level of lesion and available motor power. In general, orthoses are prescribed to support all joints around which there are paralyzed or weak muscles.

Thus, joints are protected from damage caused by weight placed on them when body parts are poorly aligned. Some children with low-level lesions may be able to stand without the benefit of braces. However, they may be doing so with their lower extremities not properly positioned, which greatly increases the chances of deformity and soft tissue damage.

An orthotist makes the braces after the child has been casted and/or measured to obtain accurate dimensions of the lower extremities. When fabrication has been completed, a session is held with the child and family to check the fit of the braces and to make any alterations that may be needed. The family receives instructions on donning the braces, precautions regarding skin care, and the types of socks and shoes to be worn.

For some children, any laced shoe is appropriate as long as the height of the heel is no more than one inch. Other children may require a high-top shoe for additional support of the ankle. High-top shoes can be purchased with a clear plastic "window" at the back of the shoe, which allows the adult to view the position of the foot or plastic brace within the shoe. Cotton knee-high socks are often recommended to be worn under the orthoses. A child with long leg plastic braces may wear tights or leotards, which decrease perspiration and irritation of the skin.

As a general rule, the child should wear the new braces for limited periods of time (approximately 1–2 hours) during the first few days. The child then has an opportunity to adjust psychologically and physically to the orthoses. Any irritation or redness of the skin should disappear within 15–20 minutes after the braces are removed. If the redness persists or blistering develops, the braces should not be worn until they are rechecked by the orthotist or physician.

Orthoses for standing are usually prescribed around the time of the first birthday, depending on the child's level of activity. Standing can be accomplished through the use of a standing brace, parapodium, or long-leg braces with pelvic band and trunk corset. In the case of the more active child who has the potential to crawl in the quadruped position and pull up to standing, braces may not be ordered until the child attempts to stand. This child usually requires less bracing than a less active child. At any rate, a program of standing in braces should certainly be initiated before the child's second birthday.

Although braces are initially prescribed to protect weakened or paralyzed areas of the body, there may be an option for less bracing in the future. As the child gains muscular strength and greater stability around joints through gross motor activities, the need for external support may decrease. Consequently, the child who once needed long-leg braces may one day need only short-leg braces. Of course, reduction in bracing can be an option only if the child gains adequate strength and joint stability. Joints surrounded by markedly weakened or paralyzed muscles must always be protected by braces if they are to bear body weight.

Ambulatory Status of the Child

For many children with myelomeningocele, ambulation becomes more difficult as they get older due to increased height and weight. Obviously, the greater the degree of paralysis, the more challenging ambulation will be at any age. Children with a high-level lesion may walk with ambulatory devices when young, but later may not, as walking becomes more demanding. By the mid-teens, many youths prefer to use a wheelchair rather than to walk with braces. This shift in mode of locomotion often occurs in early adolescence (Carroll, 1983).

The eventual ambulatory status of a child is predicted in part by the level of the paralysis. Bleck (1975) has suggested that use of a wheelchair is associated with a lesion above the twelfth thoracic level; partial household ambulation with braces and crutches is related to a lesion between the twelfth thoracic and fourth lumbar level; and community ambulation with assistive devices is common with a lesion from the fourth lumbar to the second sacral level (see Appendix A).

Findley (1983) has suggested that mobility as a young child is a better predictor of adolescent function than is the level of lesion. In his study, children who did not walk outside independently by 6 years of age did not ambulate at all as adolescents. Children who began walking outside between 4 and 6 years of age, or earlier, both walked and used a wheelchair as teenagers. Other children in the study solely used ambulation.

In addition to level of lesion, available muscle power, and history of early motor development, there are other factors that contribute to the eventual ambulatory status of the individual. These considerations include the extent of orthopaedic deformities; such factors as spasticity, age, obesity, and level of motivation; periods of immobilization (due to surgery, illness, or problems with bracing); and the individual's walking speed and physical endurance.

For many families, it is helpful to introduce early the concept that functional independence for the child may best be achieved by a combination of wheelchair use and ambulation with braces. On different occasions, one mode of locomotion may be preferred over the other. For example, the wheelchair may be more functional for use in a crowded shopping mall or for traveling long distances outdoors. This approach avoids the narrow attitude that ambulation is always the desired means of mobility.

Types of Braces

Standing Brace   The standing brace gives maximum support to the child's trunk and lower extremities to allow for early standing (see Figure 5.2). It is most useful for the child with a high-level lesion who has difficulty keeping the trunk erect.

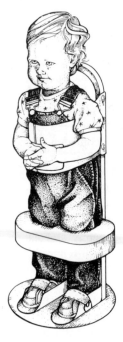

Figure 5.2.   Child in a standing brace.

Advantages   Since it is fabricated from a kit and assembled at the time of fitting, the standing brace is simple, less expensive, and fitted more quickly than other types of orthoses.

Disadvantages   Since it is generally prefabricated, the standing brace allows for little adjustment to fit the specific needs of the individual child. The brace is limited to standing; it must be removed in order for the child to sit.

Parapodium   The parapodium also provides maximum support to the trunk and legs for early standing (see Figure 5.3). It can be worn when the child is sitting or standing. The wide base allows the child to stand independently without hand support. Ambulation can be achieved through a twisting side-to-side action of the upper body, or the parapodium can be used with crutches for a swing-type gait. A special footplate platform can be attached to some parapodiums to create a swivel walker. In this device, the child can locomote without the need of other aids by rocking the trunk from side to side to propel the footplates forward in steplike fashion.

Advantages   The standard parapodium allows the child to stand and locomote without hand support. It allows the child to sit while in the orthosis.

Disadvantages   Since the standard parapodium does not require use of the hands, the child does not practice standing with crutches, which is required in ambulating with long-leg braces. Also, the rocking or twisting pattern of

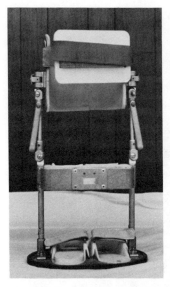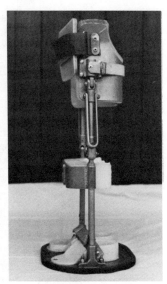

Figure 5.3. Standard parapodium, front and side views.

ambulation that the child learns to use may interfere with developing a more desirable swing-through or reciprocal gait pattern at a later date.

The parapodium is seldom used past the early childhood years since it is a high energy–consuming, slow form of locomotion requiring a level floor. Also, from a cosmetic point of view, it requires an unusual gait pattern that older children tend to resist.

Long-Leg Braces with Pelvic Band   As illustrated in Figure 5.4, long-leg braces give support below the waist and can be fitted with a corset attachment for trunk support if necessary. Although traditionally made of stainless steel uprights with a leather pelvic band, and thigh and calf cuffs, long-leg braces are now usually made of aluminum uprights and plastic cuffs to decrease their weight.

Advantages   Long-leg braces are individually fitted to the needs of the child and allow for greater adjustment for growth. The orthotic joints can be unlocked for sitting and for ambulation training if desired. Aluminum and plastic braces are lightweight for greater ease in moving and can be fitted with many styles of shoes.

Disadvantages   The child must use arm support or be placed in a standing table in order to maintain the upright position.

Short-Leg Braces   Short-leg braces are worn below the knee to give support to the foot and ankle. They are either made of metal with leather calf cuffs that fit into the heel of a special shoe, or they are a plastic mold that surrounds the back of the leg and bottom of the foot and inserts into a regular

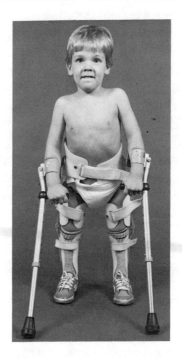

Figure 5.4. Child in long-leg braces with pelvic band, and Lofstrand crutches.

may cause an abnormal force at the knees (which are frequently unstable in the shoe (see Figure 5.5). These braces are suitable for the child who has good strength and stability at the hips and knees. Ambulation may be accomplished with or without additional assistive aids. Short-leg braces can also be used as positioning devices to maintain alignment of the feet.

Advantages   Short-leg braces are less cumbersome than the braces previously mentioned, since the child needs a minimum degree of support. Since the plastic braces provide direct contact with the calf, ankle, and foot, they maintain optimum alignment. The plastic braces are also lighter and allow for wear with different shoes, including sneakers.

Disadvantages   Since plastic braces have more surface contact, the child's feet tend to perspire. There is also a greater propensity for skin breakdown if the braces are improperly fitted. Short-leg braces do not control rotation at the hips, which may cause the feet to point in or out.

Internal or external rotation at the hip causing the feet to turn in or out may be controlled by twister cables attached from the short-leg braces to a pelvic band. Caution is in order when recommending twisters, however, because they

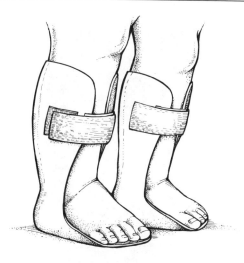

Figure 5.5. Plastic short-leg braces.

child with myelomeningocele). An alternative approach to controlling rotation at the hips is the use of metal uprights between the short-leg braces and the pelvic band.

Craig-Scott Brace The Craig-Scott long-leg brace offers a three-point pressure system that allows the child with high-level paraplegia to stand and ambulate with a minimum of support. The counterpressure system maintains the hip and knee in extension and stabilizes the ankle. Designed primarily for individuals with traumatic spinal cord injuries, these braces have been used with children with myelomeningocele when modified with a pelvic band and a "butterfly" attachment to control the position of the pelvis. Because of the added weight at the base of these braces, standing can be maintained without hand support and ambulation with crutches is made easier by the "pendulum-type" swing-through gait that is employed.

Advantages The Craig-Scott brace may allow the child with a high-level lesion to ambulate more easily. Also, it does not require hand support to maintain standing.

Disadvantages The brace is expensive and has no adjustment to allow for growth.

Reciprocating Hip Extension Brace This long-leg brace is specially designed to enhance a reciprocal gait pattern (see Figure 5.6). A cable mechanism decreases the tendency of the child to assume hip flexion when standing. To ambulate with an assistive device, the child advances one leg in flexion while the cable extends the opposite hip.

Advantages The reciprocating gait orthosis is most successful if the

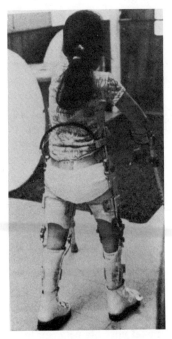

Figure 5.6.   Child in reciprocating hip extension brace. (From Molnar, G.E. [1985]. *Pediatric rehabilitation* [p. 194]. Baltimore: Williams & Wilkins; reprinted by permission.)

child has strong hip flexors. Its construction accommodates for weak hip extensors. A cable release allows the child to sit when wearing the brace.

   Disadvantages   The child usually does not progress beyond household ambulation with this orthosis.

OTHER MOBILITY AIDS

Gross motor activities such as rolling, belly crawling, quadrupedal crawling, and walking promote the acquisition of skills in all developmental areas. For example, movement activities increase muscle strength, coordination, perception, and body awareness while providing an opportunity for environmental exploration. Having a means of independent, functional locomotion is important for the physical, social, and emotional development of the child.

   Because of specific muscle paralysis and weakness, the child with spina bifida may be delayed in the development of gross motor skills or may require assistance to accomplish them. It is essential to provide the child with a variety of activities that encourage mobility. Activities need to be realistically achievable while simultaneously providing a challenge. Help is offered only as necessary in order to promote independence. It is often more time consuming to allow the child to complete a task in a self-reliant fashion, but such an experience instills a sense of physical and emotional competence.

Equipment can be purchased, adapted, or fabricated to assist the child with independent mobility. A scooter board can be propelled solely by use of the arms. Tricycles are appropriate for children who have adequate muscle strength in the legs. Tricycles can be adapted with footstraps on the pedals and trunk supports to aid sitting balance. Special hand-propelled tricycles and other riding toys are also available. A child who has total paralysis of the legs but good strength in the arms can ride such a tricycle. These low-to-the-ground riding toys and go-carts are also useful for early training in wheelchair mobility.

Some toddlers and preschool children are most independent in a wheel-chair, while others may walk with braces and an assistive device. Rollators and walkers provide greater standing balance and support than crutches. However, they cannot be maneuvered as easily and safely as crutches over uneven surfaces such as steps, gravel, or grass. The handles of the walker or rollator can be turned up so that the child grips them with the wrists in neutral alignment and the forearms in midposition (see Figure 5.7). This adaptation is indicated when the child tends to exhibit excessive flexion and ulnar deviation of the wrists when gripping the handles (i.e., the wrists are bent outward in the direction of the little finger). When possible, a child should begin ambulation training on crutches to avoid the necessity for retraining when changing from the walker or rollator to crutches.

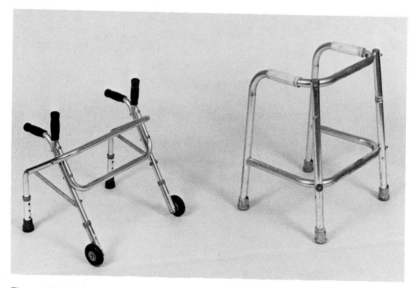

Figure 5.7. Rollator with turned up handles (left) and a walker (right).

The two major types of crutches are axillary crutches, which fit into the axilla (armpit), and Lofstrand crutches, which attach to the forearm (see Figure 5.4). Lofstrand crutches are preferred for children who will require long-term use. Children tend to lean on axillary crutches, which places undue pressure on the armpits and can cause nerve damage. Forearm crutches avoid this risk. Crutches and other assistive devices have rubber tips on the base to prevent slipping. These tips should be checked periodically for wear and replaced as needed. Likewise, nuts and screws on any orthopaedic appliance should be occasionally checked to ensure a tight fit.

Particularly during periods of marked linear growth, it is important to monitor the height of the child's assistive devices. An incorrect height can make ambulation difficult or dangerous. A therapist can adjust the size of the equipment if it is inappropriate. When holding the handles of the walker, rollator, or crutches in erect standing, the child's elbows should be bent at a 30-degree angle of flexion. Generally, the handles are at the level of the greater trochanter of the femur (the most prominent bony landmark on the lateral aspect of the hip). This height facilitates maximal use of the arms for strength. If axillary crutches are employed, the top of the crutch should rest 2–3 inches below the child's armpit so that there is less of a tendency to lean on the crutches while standing.

◇ CHAPTER 6 ◇

Perceptual-Motor Performance

PERCEPTUAL-MOTOR PERFORMANCE INVOLVES THE ABILITY TO RECEIVE, INtegrate, and organize sensory stimuli in a manner that allows for the planning and execution of purposeful movement. As Chapter 2 discusses, children with spina bifida may have deficits in sensory, perceptual, and/or cognitive processing that affect their motor competence. This chapter presents strategies and activities to promote the development of ocular-motor skills, visual perception, somatosensory perception, and fine motor coordination.

OCULAR-MOTOR SKILLS

Children with spina bifida may have visual impairments, such as diminished acuity (refractive errors), nystagmus, or strabismus, requiring the services of an ophthalmologist or optometrist. It is important, however, for early intervention and preschool programs to conduct their own assessment of the child's functional vision in order to determine: 1) the impact of the child's visual status on daily performance, and 2) intervention strategies that will encourage the development and use of visual skills.

A comprehensive protocol for evaluating functional vision has been described by Langley (1980). Although this test instrument is designed for multiply handicapped individuals, it is useful in the assessment of young children in such areas as awareness of visual stimuli, ocular-motor control, vision at near and far distances, and peripheral field vision. The STYCAR test is another instrument appropriate for this population (Sheridan, 1973).

When assessing ocular-motor skills or providing intervention, the physical environment should be structured to elicit the child's maximum visual performance. In general, a diffuse light is preferred, so that the work area is no more illuminated than the rest of the room. Often classroom and clinic settings are overly bright, resulting in glare and visual fatigue. The degree of illumination can be controlled by a rheostat on the light fixtures and venetian blinds on the windows. Direct, glaring sunlight can be avoided by adjusting the blinds to reflect the light off the ceiling. If fluorescent lighting is used, the "daylight" or "warmlight" fluorescent tubes are recommended for a soft quality of illumination. Fluorescent fixtures should be covered with diffusing screens to prevent glare.

The amount of illumination can be adapted to meet special needs. Some children with poor acuity or visual attention may respond best in a partially darkened room with illuminated toys. During regular programming, the lights can be temporarily dimmed to achieve a calming influence on overly stimulated young children.

Consideration should also be given to limiting distractions in the environment. The room should be free of clutter, distracting pictures on the wall, and extraneous noise. The floor or table surface on which the child performs activities should offer a high level of contrast to the materials. All work surfaces should be nonreflecting to avoid glare.

A variety of materials can be utilized that are well suited to the age and visual development of the child. Familiar or novel toys can be chosen depending on which type the child finds particularly motivating. Often young children prefer brightly colored objects, patterned stimuli, and toys that offer multisensory experiences (e.g., experiences that combine texture, sound, and movement). Orange, red, and yellow are visually stimulating colors. Black and yellow present a sharp contrast. Effective stimuli for eliciting and maintaining visual responses in infants or children with poor visual attention include: the human face, plastic Slinky, shiny pinwheels, mechanical spinning toys, and plastic "Sesame Street" finger puppets illuminated by a penlight. The commercially available materials developed by the Johnson and Johnson Baby Products Company have particular visual attraction for most infants.

Since young children may lose interest in a toy quickly, it is wise to have several available for working on each ocular-motor skill. Initially, it may be necessary to pair an auditory stimulus with the visual stimulus in order to elicit visual attending. For example, one can use a colorful squeeze toy that emits a noise. Some children exhibit delays in responding. Therefore, the child should be exposed to several trials and allowed a latency period from the time the stimulus is presented to the time a response can be produced.

Depending on the age of the child, ocular-motor skills can be assessed in a supine, prone, or sitting position. An infant can be placed in a semireclined posture in an infant seat, whereas the older child is most functional in supported or independent sitting. The practitioner should keep in mind that the quality of ocular skills can vary depending on the physical position. For instance, a child may have poorer visual localization and tracking when in an antigravity position requiring greater postural control.

During assessment and subsequent intervention, the child should be in a secure, symmetrical position. Proximal stability of the head and trunk is a prerequisite for optimal ocular-motor performance. Guidelines for proper positioning, such as those that Chapters 3 and 5 describe, should be followed. An abnormal postural pattern can undermine visual abilities. For example, extensor arching of the head and trunk may cause the eyes to deviate upward under the influence of the tonic labyrinthine reflex. It is then difficult for the child to locate and follow objects in the environment. If a child with multiple handicaps has a dominant asymmetrical tonic neck reflex, the eyes may deviate in the direction of the rotated head. The child may then be unable to track visually to the body midline or past it to the other side.

Some children with spina bifida may tend to sit in a slumped posture. The pelvis assumes a posterior tilt that causes rounding of the spine. With the trunk and neck flexed, these children hyperextend the head at the atlanto-occipital joint in order to observe the surroundings. That is, the cervical neck is flexed and the head is poked up using extension. In this position, skills in visual and auditory tracking are limited. The child does not have the weight shift and rotation of the trunk that are required for postural adjustment in attending to the environment.

If the child is posturally insecure, there will be a tendency to tense the muscles in order to gain stability. These tensing patterns may include: elevation of the shoulder girdle, adduction (retraction) of the scapulae, posturing of the arms against the trunk with shoulder hyperextension and elbow flexion, and fisting of the hands. This increase in muscular tension indicates that the child's position should be modified to improve proximal stability and thus, visual-motor competence. External support may be required through adaptation of the furniture, the use of a seatbelt, or other modifications.

The professional literature has described activities to promote visual skills (Langley, 1980; Robinson & Robinson, 1978; Smith & Cote, 1982). Of particular importance is the ability of both eyes to work together in a coordinated fashion (i.e., conjugate vision). As Chapter 2 discusses, strabismus is a common ocular problem requiring medical attention in children with spina bifida. Strabismus may affect the child's visual functioning by impairing general ocular movements, depth perception, and convergence (directing both eyes to focus on a near point).

The following section discusses facilitating ocular-motor abilities in the areas of visual fixation, shift of gaze, tracking, and scanning.

Visual Fixation

Visual fixation is the ability to direct the eyes to the same point in space for a period of time. The gaze is such that the image of the stimulus falls on the fovea centralis (the depression in the macula of the retina, which provides the most acute vision). Fixation is a prerequisite skill for other ocular-motor responses such as shifting gaze between objects or tracking.

Sample Activities to Promote Visual Fixation

1. With the child well positioned with the head and trunk in midline, the adult presents a brightly colored object 10–12 inches from the face. The adult shakes the toy to attract the child's visual attention. A reflection of the stimulus on the child's pupils is an indicator of fixation.
2. The adult flashes a penlight that is placed inside a finger puppet to the left of the child. The child is allowed to fixate visually on the puppet for a few seconds. Then the adult turns the penlight off and moves the puppet 3 inches toward the child's midline. The penlight is blinked on again and the child is allowed to achieve fixation on the puppet. The adult repeats this on-and-off sequence as he or she progresses the stimulus to the right side of the child's visual field. Depending on the child's skill, this activity can be conducted in a horizontal, vertical, or diagonal direction.

Shift of Gaze

Shift of gaze (or alternating gaze) is the ability to change fixation from one object to another. It is a precursor to scanning abilities. In these activities, the adult notes whether the child shifts spontaneously or whether shaking or sound cues are required. If shifting does not occur without cues, the child will be "stimulus controlled" and have difficulty attending to relevant stimuli. The child should be able to shift gaze easily between two toys four or five times in a 5-second period.

Sample Activities to Promote Shift of Gaze

1. The child is encouraged to look alternately at two objects the same distance away. The toys should be identical in interest and size, such as puppets or spinner toys. The adult presents the two objects about 12 inches away from the child's eyes on a horizontal plane and approximately 2–4 inches apart. The adult should observe if the child spontaneously shifts gaze from one object to the other. If this does not occur, the adult obtains visual fixation on the first object by shaking it. When fixation is achieved, the adult facilitates shifting of gaze to the other object by shaking or activating it. This sequence is repeated, allowing several seconds of attending before attracting attention to the other item.

    This activity can be graded in complexity by gradually increasing the distance between the two objects. The child first practices the skill with the toys on a horizontal plane before being required to shift gaze vertically or diagonally. To increase interest, hand puppets activated by the adult can conduct a conversation with each other and with the child.
2. The adult presents two differently colored penlights in front of the child, approximately 4 inches apart. The adult turns one of the penlights on and has the child visually attend for 3 seconds. Then that light is turned off and

the other penlight is activated. The adult continues this alternating sequence. The space between the two lights is gradually increased and their position is altered so as to require horizontal, vertical, or diagonal eye movements. This task can be made easier by the adult slightly darkening the room to increase the contrast between the flashlight and the environmental illumination.

Visual Tracking

Visual tracking is the ability to follow moving objects with the eyes. This skill assists the infant in developing the concepts of object permanence and object constancy (Blackwell, Britz, Jans, Rock, & Vedovatti, 1981). Care should be taken that tracking skills are age appropriate in prone or supine lying as well as sitting. In general, however, an upright position is preferred for intervention. The young child can recline in an infant seat, the older child can sit on the floor or on a chair. If the child has poor head control, the supine position on the floor or wedge can be modified with cushions to achieve partial head and hip flexion.

The first eye movements to track objects generally occur in the horizontal plane, with the eyes and head moving as a unit. As head control in the midline develops, the infant begins to isolate movements of the eyes while the head remains in a stable position. Like gaze shifting, controlled tracking skills progress in a developmental pattern—from horizontal eye movements to eye movements in a vertical, diagonal, and circular direction. Activities to encourage tracking should thus be graded in this sequence.

Sample Activities to Promote Visual Tracking

1. The child should be encouraged to track faces, brightly lit objects, and toys. The adult presents the object at the child's midline, slightly below eye level, and at a distance of 8–12 inches. When fixation on the object is obtained, the adult moves the object slowly to one side to have the child follow it. The adult should begin moving the object in small arcs (e.g., 45 degrees from the midline), progressing to a full 180-degree arc. The object should be moved at a standard distance from the child's face. That is, the object should be moved in an arc that ensures that the distance from the nose is constant. The reason is that movement of the object in a straight line complicates the task by requiring adjustment of the eyes to accommodate for changes in distance (i.e., modifications in convergence).

   Care should also be taken to move the toy very slowly across the midline when going from one side to the other, since crossing the midline with the eyes is initially difficult for some children. In the young infant, fixation on a toy to elicit tracking may be most easily obtained if the object is first presented from the side. In this case, the adult should have the infant practice tracking from the side toward the midline as an initial step.

When the child successfully tracks in a horizontal plane, similar activities are introduced to obtain tracking in vertical and diagonal planes, and finally in a circular pattern. To encourage tracking in a circle, the child first fixates on a toy, then the object is moved in a circle approximately 12 inches in diameter. The diameter of the circle is gradually increased in size. It is important to note that the child will have to turn the head in combination with the eyes as the arc of movement increases.

Downward gaze may initially require flexion of the head and neck to view an object. When head control is poor and chin tucking is not achieved, vertical tracking can be practiced while the child is assisted in stabilizing the head in midline. The adult presents a toy slightly below eye level and slowly moves it downward and then back up to eye level. Vertical tracking above eye level can sometimes elicit an increase in extensor posturing in children with abnormal muscle tone. Changes in muscle tone should be monitored during activities requiring upward gaze so that positioning and handling can be altered as needed to inhibit abnormal postures.

2. The adult inserts a brightly colored ball in a clear plastic tube positioned horizontally at eye level in front of the child. By tilting the tube slightly, the ball will roll from one end of the cylinder to the other and thus elicit visual tracking by the child. This game can be graded in complexity by decreasing the size of the ball and varying its color (a neutral-colored ball provides less contrast and is therefore more difficult to follow). The direction of tracking is varied by the degree of tilt of the cylinder.

Another game is to use a partially covered tube to encourage visual anticipation of the reappearance of an object. The ball is inserted at one end of the tube, and the child's attention is drawn to the reappearance of the ball at the other end of the tube. With repetition, the child is able to track and shift gaze quickly from one end of the cylinder to the other in anticipation of the ball's appearance.

Other play activities to encourage tracking include: following balls of various sizes as they are rolled across the floor or table; following a pull toy or a truck as it is moved; and observing the fall of objects that are slowly poured from a container onto a surface.

3. Activities to improve tracking skills in the toddler and preschool-age child are frequently most successful when the child is involved as an active participant. Horizontal tracking can be encouraged by having the child push a car along a "road" that has been drawn across a table or along a strip of masking tape on the floor. On a chalkboard, the child can trace over simple chalk lines with a finger in order to erase them. The child can start with horizontal chalk lines and progress to vertical, diagonal, and circular lines. For the child who is able to manage a piece of chalk, the white lines can be traced with colored chalk. To maintain the child's interest, these

chalkboard games can be integrated into a story in which the child follows a map in order to travel from home to the school or store.

Visual Scanning

Visual scanning is the ability to change visual fixation in a linear plane from one object to another and then to a third, and fourth. A prerequisite for academic-related skills is the capacity to scan in an organized manner from left to right and top to bottom. Scanning is necessary for such activities as copying and printing, reading across a line, and performing arithmetic problems. Typically, a child begins to apply these skills in the preschool and kindergarten years when preacademic work is introduced.

Sample Activities to Promote Visual Scanning

1. Three objects are placed in a row in front of the child, on a horizontal plane, a few inches apart. The child's view is blocked by a piece of cardboard held by the adult. The cardboard is then removed in a left to right progression to display the objects and encourage scanning in this direction. The task can be graded in complexity by increasing the number of objects and the speed at which the cardboard barrier is removed. Later the task can be repeated without the cardboard. Instead, each object is tapped by the adult in a left-to-right sequence.

2. A variety of fine motor games can be used to encourage visual scanning from left to right and top to bottom. Activities familiar to the child can be structured in a way that facilitates ocular movements in these directions. In playing with a pegboard, for example, the child can duplicate a line of pegs starting on the left and progressing to the right. Similarly, when stringing beads, the child can pick up a horizontal row of beads in a left-to-right progression. Blocks, picture cards, and pasting activities can also be positioned in this fashion.

VISUAL PERCEPTION

Visual perception is a complex process resulting in the ability to interpret and understand what is seen with the eyes. It is dependent on a variety of skills, including: visual acuity, the ocular-motor control necessary for moving the eyes to scan for information, and the ability to attend to what is relevant in the environment. Selective attention is necessary to focus on and discriminate details that are observed; then, the visual input has to be interpreted for its meaning. The ability to interpret what is seen is closely tied to sensory integrative processes and cognitive development.

Typically, the young child uses visual information in the current situation to assist him or her in determining the appropriate action to be taken. For example, looking at a novel or unfamiliar toy results in exploratory behavior such as mouthing, touching, or grasping, whereas a familiar toy may elicit a more purposeful action. Visual information is stored in memory for recall at a later time; the ability to relate visual stimuli to previous experience contributes to the child's growing cognitive capacity (e.g., the ability to generalize or conceptualize objects into categories).

Visual perceptual-motor integration occurs when the child combines skills in visual perception with a gross or fine motor action. Block stacking is an example of a simple visual perceptual-motor task, whereas writing is a more sophisticated task. In building a block tower, the child perceives the relationship of one block to another in a vertical position, while at the same time applying the motor control needed to place and release the blocks successfully. Writing requires visual memory of what the letters look like and the motor planning required to form the letters. In clinical practice with very young children, it is difficult to isolate visual-perceptual skills from motor activity. It is usually necessary to assess visual perception indirectly through observing the child's control of self and objects in space.

Several points should be kept in mind when assessing visual perceptual-motor skills and planning an appropriate program of intervention. These perceptual skills encompass a wide variety of competencies ranging from simple to complex. Common perceptual skills include: the recognition of part-to-whole relationships; figure-ground perception; visual memory; depth perception; discrimination of form, size, color, and position; and the recognition of similarities and differences.

The ability to understand what is seen and make use of the information in a meaningful way is dependent on combining varied processes in the brain. Ayres (1979) has emphasized the role of sensory integrative processing in the development of visual perception. Sensations from the tactile, proprioceptive, and vestibular systems are combined with visual input to obtain meaning from the visual environment. In this sense, visual perception can be viewed as an end product that is partially dependent on adequate somatosensory integration. Visual information is most meaningful when it is associated with sensory information from the other senses, such as touch and hearing. The association or pairing of sensory input allows the child to visualize objects or people when a sound is heard, or to identify an object when it is felt but not seen.

Cognition plays an important role in understanding visual information. The stages of cognitive development in the sensorimotor period (as described by Piaget, 1952) contribute essential foundations for visual perception. An example of a cognitive skill that influences perceptual development is object permanence. Object permanence is the awareness that objects have an independent existence even when they are not seen. It is demonstrated when the infant visually searches for a fallen toy or looks for hidden objects. Remembering what is seen (visual memory) is enhanced by this developing cognitive capacity. The functional use of vision is therefore related to the child's level of perceptual and cognitive processing.

Early sensory and motor experiences facilitate the development of visual perception. For example, gross and fine motor activities of the infant contribute to an appreciation of spatial relationships (that is, perception of oneself in relation to the environment and of the position of objects in relation to one another). The child learns about space by moving up and down, and by going in and out of and under and over obstacles in the environment. Such motor exploration develops the perception of one's size in relation to the external world. Through trial and error, a child also learns that some objects fit inside others or can be stacked on top of one another. In the early period of developing spatial concepts, it is common for a child to enjoy putting objects into containers and taking them out again, and to experiment with crawling into narrow openings or under tables.

There is, however, controversy as to the nature of infant perception and the specific role of motor activity in influencing its development. Research over the last 20 years has increasingly indicated that infants are capable of a variety of visual discriminations regardless of their experience with touching or manipulating objects (Cohen, DeLoache, & Strauss, 1979). This point of view is supported by the performance of many children with multiple handicaps. In spite of limited opportunity for play with objects due to impaired arm use, many children develop perceptual skills on a complex level (Kearsley, 1981). These observations suggest that motor experiences contribute to but are not mandatory for the development of visual perception.

Clinically, there is a need to understand more specifically how perception develops and what skills contribute to adequate perceptual functioning. Numerous practitioners have addressed the area of visual perception by theoretically dividing it into hypothetical parts or subskills. These approaches are useful to the clinician in understanding the components of a complex process. It should be kept in mind, however, that the child in reality perceives the environment as a whole, relating past experiences to the current situation. When observing a child, it is often difficult to determine the specific components of perception that are in operation at a given moment.

In assessing visual perceptual-motor skills, repeated observations of the child under a variety of circumstances may be necessary in an attempt to delineate the child's functional ability and learning needs. When the child has limited motor responses, alternative methods for assessing perceptual and cognitive development may be required. It may be necessary to make inferences about these areas through monitoring changes in the child's level of attention, affect, gross body movement, or habituation to presented stimuli. Various response modes for communication may be needed, such as the use of eye gaze.

Sample intervention strategies are presented in specific subskill areas to facilitate visual perceptual-motor development in these various areas. Since an in-depth discussion of visual perception is beyond the scope of this book, only the most common areas of concern for some children with spina bifida are addressed. Care is needed, however, to avoid training in isolated subskills that may have little relevance to the child's overall performance. It is important to reevaluate on a regular basis the extent to which a child is acquiring competencies that generalize to a variety of life situations.

Visual Discrimination of Color, Form, and Size

The visual discrimination of color, form, and size contributes to the child's ability to recognize and distinguish common objects. It allows identification of the specific attributes of objects. Thus, it is an important prerequisite to understanding similarities and differences in the environment and contributes to the ability to classify objects by category.

Intervention to enhance visual discrimination in the preschool population includes enabling the child to recognize such attributes as color, form, and size, then to match attributes, and finally to sort into categories. Generally, the child acquires these abilities in relation to one attribute before integrating several attributes into one activity. For example, sorting by color or shape alone precedes sorting by both color and shape (such as sorting red and blue circles and squares).

Sample Activities to Promote Visual Discrimination of Color, Form, and Size

1. In learning to discriminate on the basis of color, the child first matches like objects of the same color. Sorting tasks can then be introduced, such as placing like-colored chips into a container of the same color, beginning with two colors and progressing to three or four colors. Initially, high-contrast colors are used, such as yellow and red. Group games such as color bingo involve the recognition and matching of four or five colors.
2. Exploration of the environment through gross motor activities can be used initially with the preschool child to increase awareness of likeness and difference in form. Creeping through, crawling over, and moving around obstacles of varying shapes promotes the awareness of object form and also develops spatial and directional orientation. Throwing bean bags and balls into large geometric shapes on the floor increases an understanding of the physical boundaries of those shapes. Recognition of form is enhanced by the early use of common three-dimensional objects, such as balls and boxes, to introduce the concepts of round and square. Other activities may include visual matching games such as picture Lotto, pasting similar shapes on paper, and sorting shapes into separate containers. Later, group games can be organized in which the children are asked to identify shapes in the environment (e.g., "Where is something round?").

3. Formboards and puzzles facilitate spatial orientation at the same time that perception of form is practiced. As the child learns to match a form with its outline in a puzzle, he or she is readied for the task of orienting objects in space more skillfully. For example, the child learns to rotate a triangle with unequal sides so as to be able to fit it into a puzzle space.

Also enhanced with puzzle construction is the perception of whole-part relationships. Once the child is adept with single-piece insert puzzles, he or she can progress to puzzles in which two pieces need to be inserted to create a complete picture—that is, the pieces represent the top and bottom or right and left sides of the picture. Large magazine pictures mounted on cardboard and cut in half are useful for this purpose. In similar fashion, broken objects such as pencils or toy cars can be used to challenge the children to put the broken parts together to make a whole object.

4. The concept of the physical constancy of size is introduced by providing concrete experience in manipulating open-ended nesting pieces such as cups, bowls, and boxes. Through trial and error, the child learns that objects fit inside one another and begins to recognize the smaller and larger of two containers. Gradually, a greater number of containers, with increasingly smaller gradations, are presented so as to encourage the development of sequential ordering by size. Montessori materials such as cylinders of graded size are useful for this purpose. Balls of varying dimensions can be tossed into a basket for the child to observe which ones do or do not fit. Objects and pictures of objects, in which the child identifies bigger/smaller and longer/shorter, may be used to help the child gain an expanded awareness of the concept of size.

Spatial Relations

The perception of spatial relations includes the ability to understand such spatial concepts as in/out, up/down, over/under, in front of/behind, and right/left. An understanding of these concepts allows children to perceive where their bodies are in relation to objects as well as the position of objects in relation to each other. (The role of gross motor activities in developing awareness of one's position in space has previously been discussed.) The following table-top activities are beneficial in introducing spatial concepts to preschool children. It is suggested that concepts be introduced one at a time to avoid confusion.

Sample Activities to Promote Awareness of Spatial Relations

1. The adult and child have an open box and several common objects such as a truck, a toy animal, and a doll. In this hide-and-seek activity, the objects are placed one at a time in different orientations to the box and the child searches to find it. Care is taken to label the placement of the objects for the child once it is found. For example, "Yes, the dog is under the box."

A game of increasing difficulty is for the adult to place objects in relation to the box and have the child imitate the placement with a similar object. The adult then progresses to placing the object, removing it, and then having the child remember where to replace the object.

2. Construction or building activities are perhaps the best means through which children learn about the relationship of objects to each other. Such activities can frequently be accomplished by the child independently or with a minimal amount of adult supervision. Simple block stacking to make towers helps a child learn the concept "on top of." Such concepts as "next to," "in front of," and "behind" are applied when lining up blocks to make a road.

   Block construction is more difficult when the child must imitate or match an adult's example. Constructing a tower using one color of blocks is a simple task, whereas constructing "steps" using two colors of blocks is quite complex. The placement and matching of colored blocks on top of a design card is a similar but more sophisticated task. It requires relating concrete objects (blocks) to an abstract representation (design card).

3. An apple is placed in front of a lunchbox on a table. The child has a paper on which different objects are drawn in a variety of positions in relation to a lunchbox. The child circles the picture that matches the concrete example of the apple in front of the lunchbox. When concrete cues are no longer needed, the child performs the task using a stimulus card with a picture. Difficulty is increased by using abstract or geometric designs instead of pictures and by decreasing the degree of positional difference.

4. Language related to spatial concepts should be emphasized. Concept labeling is introduced as the child begins to demonstrate awareness of the position of objects in space during gross motor and manipulative activities. The adult describes relationships for the child ("The snack is *on* the table") and provides verbal directions for simple tasks ("Put both hands *around* the ball"). A large circle is created on the floor using masking tape. During group activities, the children are asked to sit on, inside, or outside the circle.

Figure-Ground Perception

Figure-ground perception is the ability to focus on relevant details in the visual environment. Figure-ground relationships provide the basis for selective attention. Those aspects of the environment being attended to become foreground, while the remaining aspects fade into background. The child demonstrates figure-ground perception when finding a favorite toy in a toy box, pointing to objects in a picture book, or locating a familiar adult in a group of people. Figure-ground perception is required in the preschool class in order to attend to the teacher and successfully perform preacademic readiness activities. Some children with spina bifida have difficulty achieving and maintaining this aspect of visual perception.

To develop figure-ground perception, activities are presented that involve the introduction of increasingly complex visual fields. The child is required to attend to the relevant stimuli despite the distracting background. The following sample activities to promote figure-ground perception are appropriate during the preschool years.

Sample Activities to Promote Figure-Ground Perception

1. The adult places chips of various colors in a box and asks the child to pick out specific colors. Note that color recognition is a prerequisite skill for this activity. Beads, blocks, or varied shapes can also be used.
2. On a large sheet of paper, the adult makes a design of overlapping yarn of three different colors. The child traces one color of yarn at a time with a finger or some hand-held object, such as a car. This activity is graded in difficulty by increasing the number of colors and the complexity of the design. A variation of this task is for the child to trace over colored, intersecting lines drawn on a piece of paper.
3. Pen-and-paper activities with hidden figures are appropriate for children who are able to trace. The child is presented with a sample picture of a form or object that is "hidden" in a distracting background. The child finds the shape in the picture and traces it. When the child recognizes forms with ease, all the objects in a picture that are the same shape are traced. For example, if the shape to be found is a circle, the child traces all the circular buttons on a picture of a child wearing a coat. To make the task more challenging, the child is requested to find shapes or objects when only a portion of the item is visible. For instance, the child finds a banana within a picture of a bowl of fruit. These activities are also helpful in reinforcing form discrimination.

Visual Memory

Visual memory is the ability to recall what has been seen in terms of its shape, color, and other relevant features. Children who have difficulty attending or who are highly distractible may benefit from a structured program that focuses on visual memory.

Sample Activities to Promote Visual Memory

1. Two different objects are presented to the child. After 30 seconds, they are covered by a cloth or a piece of cardboard and one object is removed. When the cover is lifted, the child identifies the object that is missing. This activity is graded by increasing the number of objects presented and decreasing the viewing time.
2. The child is presented with a variety of objects or pictures and is briefly shown one matching object or picture. When that object is removed from sight, the child finds its match from the assortment.

3. Visual memory tasks can easily be incorporated into a prewriting program. The child is shown a sample of a horizontal, vertical, or diagonal line. After viewing the line for several seconds, the child duplicates the line on a piece of paper. Or the child and adult both have a picture of an outline of a face. The adult draws one facial feature on his or her outline and lets the child view it for 5 seconds. The child then draws the same part on his or her outline. The process continues until a whole face or human form is drawn. The activity is graded by increasing or decreasing the viewing time or by drawing two parts at a time.

4. Visual memory can also be fostered by the daily routine of the classroom or home. During or after a group "show-and-tell" time, the teacher can review what each child brought to share by asking questions ("What did Bobby bring?" or "Who showed us the doll?").

SOMATOSENSORY PERCEPTION

Somatosensory perception refers to the integration of vestibular, tactile, and/or proprioceptive sensation. These body senses provide information about the child's internal environment. Somatosensory perception is important because it contributes to the development of a body scheme and motor planning. Body scheme is the inner awareness of one's body parts, the relationship of these parts to the body as a whole, and how the parts move through space. It is the brain's unconscious mental picture of the body. Chapter 2 describes the difficulties in sensory processing of some children with spina bifida, which may interfere with learning. These problems include movement and tactile defensiveness and poor tactile discrimination in the upper limbs. This section discusses intervention to promote vestibular, tactile, and proprioceptive integration.

Vestibular Processing

The vestibular system is involved in the sensation of movement. Its sensory receptors, located in the labyrinths of the inner ear, include the semicircular canals, which detect changes in the head's position, and the otoliths, which respond to the pull of gravity. In the developing child, adequate processing of movement sensation by the vestibular system has an influence on a wide variety of functions. Among the most important of these functions are muscle tone, postural control, balance, and ocular-motor skills. The vestibular system has a critical role in facilitating the brain's capacity for sensory integration.

Many children with myelomeningocele are fearful of movement because of their physical paralysis. When a motor handicap interferes with reactions that maintain balance in upright positions and prevent falling, it is understandable that the child may be fearful during independent movement or when being moved. These children frequently have the ability to receive and interpret movement sensations but lack the motor skills to respond adequately to a change in their center of gravity. The gross motor activities described in Chapter 3 and 9 are appropriate for children whose fear of movement arises from a motor deficit.

It is important for all children in the early years to experience movement that provides sensory input to the vestibular system. However, it should be kept in mind that movement can be a powerful source of sensory input. An activity that provides excessive movement can be overstimulating and result in sensory overload and disorganization. Signs of overstimulation in the child include an increase in activity level or overarousal after the movement has been stopped, dizziness, and nausea. An unusual amount of perspiration and an increase in heart rate may also be noted. On the other hand, certain types of movement, particularly those that are slow, rhythmic, and repetitive, can result in over-inhibition or a slowing down of the nervous system. Overinhibition results in a decrease in heart rate and respiration, yawning, or lethargy. Motor activities should be immediately stopped at signs of either extreme reaction.

Two important guidelines are used to guard against either overstimulation or overinhibition resulting from inappropriate motor activity. First, the child should initiate the motor experience. The adult provides the environment and the opportunity for movement that will allow the child to be an active participant. The child is given encouragement and assistance but is not forced to participate in an activity if fearful or resistant. Second, it must be kept in mind that the child is the best regulator of the proper intensity of the sensory input. Thus, an activity is terminated when the child indicates that the level of tolerance has been reached. Most children will stop an activity on their own prior to overstimulation.

Occasionally, a therapeutic evaluation of the child with spina bifida will indicate a specific problem in processing the sensation of movement through the vestibular system. In such cases, a therapist may incorporate movement-oriented experiences within the intervention, such as swinging, rotation, and quick accelerations and decelerations in linear movement. This type of stimulation requires close monitoring of the child's responses and is most appropriately applied by a clinician skilled in the use of a sensory-integrative approach to treatment (Ayres, 1979).

Tactile and Proprioceptive Processing

Intervention should include activities to foster the perceptual processing of tactile and proprioceptive information. The skin has specialized receptors that are sensitive to touch, pressure, cold, warmth, and pain. Other receptors are located in the muscles, tendons, and joints. These proprioceptors provide an appreciation of the position of body parts at any moment in time. Thus, one is aware of the body's position at rest as well as during movement. This awareness of joint motion is sometimes referred to as kinesthesia.

A specially designated area for sensory-oriented play is one of the best ways to incorporate sensory activities into the overall program. This area is designed to provide experiences in substance play (sand, water, clay, Play-Doh, fingerpaints), as well as opportunities to explore the sensory attributes of objects. Suggested play materials include:

1. Texture boards ranging from soft to coarse (e.g., fur, cotton, corduroy, wool, sandpaper). Scraps of the same textures can be used to encourage matching of textures. When the child is familiar with matching using both touch and vision, he or she is encouraged to match with eyes closed, using touch alone.
2. A plastic washbasin filled with uncooked rice, beans, or pasta. The child can search for toys or shapes hidden in the rice, by looking or not looking.
3. A "feely box" containing a variety of common objects. The child can describe objects that are being felt or can match objects in the box to similar objects on the table.
4. A scrap box of cloth, felt, paper, yarn, string, and macaroni for arts and crafts activities such as making collages.
5. Tactile books, which provide items of different textures for the child to feel.

Sample Activities to Promote Tactile Discrimination

1. The children rub body parts with powder, lotion, or cloth of different textures. The adult reinforces sensory awareness of the body by discussing what it feels like. If a child is tactually defensive, it is advisable to begin rubbing with deep pressure parts of the body that will be least likely to elicit an aversive response. Generally, the hands are least defensive, followed by the arms and legs. The face, neck, soles of the feet, and front of the trunk are usually the most sensitive body parts.
2. The adult places a common object or shape in a large bag. The children take turns reaching in the bag without looking, to feel and then identify the object. A variation of the activity is to place a small object (such as a marble, penny, or crayon) in the child's hand. The child identifies the object by touch with the eyes closed.
3. Fingerpainting, with sand or uncooked rice added to vary the texture of the paint.
4. Tracking activities on sandpaper, corrugated cardboard, or a textured board.

A child's awareness of joint position develops primarily through weight-bearing experiences on the arms and legs. Some children with spina bifida may require special programming to increase proprioceptive awareness in the arms. Decreased proprioceptive discrimination may be due to limited motor experiences in weight-bearing postures or to a deficit in sensory integrative development. Weight bearing on the arms can be incorporated into gym and gross motor activities as described in Chapters 3 and 9.

Sample Activities to Promote Proprioceptive Awareness

1. "Simon Says" game. Initially, the adult demonstrates arm movement while also giving verbal cues, and the children imitate these movements. When the movements are imitated accurately, the children are encouraged to make the movements with eyes closed, relying solely on verbal cues. For example, "Put your hands on your head"; "Reach up with your elbows straight"; "Make your arms go round and round in a big circle." Variations of Simon Says can include discriminating between fast and slow movements: "Shake your hands as fast as you can"; "Shake your hands very slowly." Performing movements while holding weights (small cans, bean bags, or wooden blocks) provides additional sensory input for discriminating limb position during movement.

2. A balloon, an 8-inch foam ball, and an 8-inch plastic ball are alternately tossed in a circle of children. The children attempt to keep the object in the air by batting it with their hands. This activity provides an opportunity for the children to feel differences in how they move their arms in response to the varying weight of the object.

3. Musical toys, finger plays, action songs, and clapping hands at a rate set by the adult assist the children to develop a sense of timing and rhythm.

4. The children take turns hammering wooden nails into a play workbench. They can progress to hammering real nails that have been previously hammered halfway into the wood. The weight of the hammer and the resistance offered by the nails provide increased proprioceptive input to the upper extremities.

A comprehensive program of sensory discrimination may also include activities to develop perception of smell, taste, and temperature. Intervention starts at a level of developing gross awareness of the sense before progressing to discrimination of pleasant and unpleasant odors, cold and warm temperatures, and sweet and sour foods. Snack time provides an opportunity for the children to experience these sensations and their related concepts within a natural context. Children who are tactually defensive, however, may demonstrate aversive responses to the smell and taste of specific foods. With these children, intervention is initially graded to avoid extreme odors and tastes, and very cold temperatures. Highly textured foods may also have to be avoided.

FINE MOTOR COORDINATION

Fine motor skills require the child to reach, grasp, and release objects in an infinite variety of coordinated movement patterns. The primary role of the arm is to position the hand so that the latter can engage in manipulation. As the term "eye-hand coordination" implies, vision is critically important in directing and grading movements of the upper extremities. However, tactile and proprioceptive information from the skin, muscles, tendons, and joints is also influential in motor planning for successful manual play.

The achievement of fine motor coordination is dependent on proximal stability of the trunk and scapula since the arm requires a firm foundation on which to move. When a child reaches for an object, postural adjustment of the head, trunk, and pelvis are often necessary to maintain balance. Similarly, the scapula slides firmly along the rib cage so that the shoulder joint is properly aligned and supported. Movements of the scapula and shoulder joint produce the motion of the arm. Consequently, strength of the scapular muscles is essential for functional reach patterns. When assessing fine motor skills, the practitioner must always remember their relationship to postural and scapular control.

An infant develops coordination of the upper extremities by assuming and maintaining antigravity positions while bearing weight on the arms. When prone lying on the elbows or extended arms, the child acquires control of the scapulae and shoulder joints by shifting the body weight in all directions. This practice is later conducted in propped sitting and quadruped.

Between 4 and 6 months, the infant develops a directed reach and gross (palmar) grasp. In this grasp pattern, the fingers press the object against the palm but the thumb does not participate. Initially, the shoulder is internally rotated and the forearm is pronated during reach. The coordination of external rotation and supination occurs gradually during the first year. By 6 months, the infant is able to engage in noisy manual play through the multisensory exploration of objects. The child enjoys vertically banging and shaking toys, and transferring them from one hand to the other.

Grasp and release activities are stressed around 7–9 months. Depending on the size of the object, the radial or thumb side of the hand becomes more active in picking up objects. At first, a radial-palmar grasp is employed, in which the item is pressed against the palm and base of the thumb. Later, a radial-digital grasp allows the object to be held between the thumb and the ends of the fingers. Greater control of wrist movement and supination are seen in handling objects and banging them together horizontally. The infant practices release by dropping and squeezing toys. Toward the end of this period, the child develops a lateral prehension, in which a small object is held between the thumb and the side of the index finger. "Poking" and "pointing" activities, with an extended index finger, begin to isolate the forefinger from the other fingers (the process of dissociation) in preparation for more sophisticated pinch patterns.

Between 10 and 12 months, the infant achieves fine prehension and controlled release. Increasingly, the wrist remains extended when grasping, and the thumb demonstrates opposition. That is, the thumb is able to rotate around for a pad-to-pad contact with the fingers. At first, a pincer grasp is used, with the thumb and index finger precisely opposing an object (two-point pinch). Later, a small object such as a pellet can be held between the tips of the thumb and forefinger (neat pincer grasp). By 12 months, the child has a controlled release and is able to put a cube into a small container. At this time, hand use is starting to differentiate so that one hand holds an object while the other manipulates it.

The Erhardt Developmental Prehension Assessment provides an in-depth description of reach and grasp skills (Erhardt, 1982). This protocol also presents the sequential development of crayon manipulation (see Figure 6.1). The child of 1–2 years initially holds the crayon with a fisted hand with the forearm slightly supinated from the midposition (palmar supinate grasp). Scribbling is accomplished predominantly with shoulder motion. In the digital pronate grasp of the 2- to 3-year-old, the forearm is pronated with all the fingers holding the crayon. Strokes are performed with the forearm and wrist moving as a unit. By 3½–4 years, the crayon is held crudely by the proximal aspect of the thumb and the index and middle fingers. In this static tripod grasp, movement occurs at the wrist with limited motion of the digits.

Gradually, between 4½ and 6 years, the mature pattern of a dynamic tripod grasp emerges. The wrist is slightly extended, the thumb opposes the distal ends of the index and middle fingers, and the ring and little finger are flexed to provide a supportive arch for the hand. The shoulder, elbow, and wrist are stabilized to allow the fingers to perform fine movements. Manipulation of the crayon occurs at the interphalangeal joints of the fingers, since the knuckles (metacarpophalangeal joints) are stable.

Competence in fine motor tasks is founded on the following major skills: postural stability, ocular-motor control, visual perception, tactile and proprioceptive discrimination, cognition, and muscular strength and coordination. As discussed in Chapter 2, children with spina bifida may have difficulties in any of these areas. Particularly in the presence of shunted hydrocephalus, the child may demonstrate poor visual-motor integration, diminished somatosensory perception, proximal and distal weakness or spasticity of the upper extremities, and inadequate establishment of hand preference. An individualized assessment is necessary to determine the child's strengths and weaknesses in the subskills required for fine motor performance. Intervention should be directed toward capitalizing on abilities while remediating deficits. The following guidelines should be considered when designing a program to enhance fine motor coordination.

Principles of Intervention

1. The child should be well positioned before engaging in activities of the upper extremity. If balance and posture are poor, the child will tend to: 1) tense the trunk and limbs to achieve artificial stability, 2) use the arms for support, or 3) resist reaching away from the body for fear of falling. The practitioner needs to monitor the degree of gross and fine motor

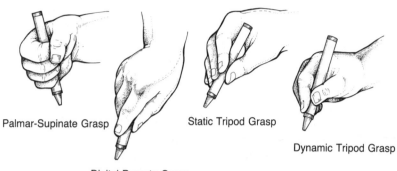

Palmar-Supinate Grasp

Static Tripod Grasp

Dynamic Tripod Grasp

Digital-Pronate Grasp

Figure 6.1. Sequential development of crayon manipulation. (Adapted from Erhardt, R. P. [1982]. *Developmental hand dysfunction: Theory, assessment, and treatment* [p. 112]. Laurel, MD: Ramsco; reprinted by permission.)

control required by the task. If the activity demands fine manipulation, external support may be necessary to ensure adequate balance. Symmetrical alignment of the body in properly fitted furniture pre-positions the child for success.

2. Since the development of antigravity postural control progresses in a proximal to distal direction, movements of the shoulder may need to be emphasized before coordination of the wrist and hand. Strengthening the muscles of the upper trunk and scapulae provides the proximal base for discrete distal movement of the limbs. (Chapter 3 offers numerous suggestions for achieving this goal.) Gross motor activities while the child is propped on one or both arms stimulate maintained contractions of the muscles. These weight-bearing tasks should be practiced with the shoulder in varying degrees of flexion.

3. In a sitting position, it is easier to reach forward or to the side than overhead or behind the body. An overhead reach requires a secure trunk to maintain balance and scapular stability to support the raised arm. To reach behind the body, the child must rotate the head and trunk while visually directing the arm backward. Usually, body weight is shifted onto one buttock as righting reactions are elicited to prevent a fall. The abdominal muscles are particularly important to maintain the trunk control necessary for reach of the arm.

    More sophisticated reach patterns can be promoted by encouraging reaching in a developmental sequence: first forward, then sideways, and finally overhead or backward. As the child acquires motor skill, toys can be positioned to facilitate reach in all directions and across the midline of the body. Of course, a child with a high-level lesion may have limitations in the more difficult reach patterns due to lack of muscle innervation of the trunk.

4. The work surface can be graded from horizontal to an incline and later to a vertical orientation. By gradually increasing the incline of a table top, the amount of support given to the child's shoulder and forearm is correspondingly decreased. More muscle action is then required to maintain the arms in an antigravity position. Educational tasks can be adapted to use of a large vertical mirror, felt board, easel, or paper taped to the wall. In this way, the child plays with both arms held in shoulder flexion away from the body. Or one arm can prop forward against the upright work surface while the other arm is engaged in the activity.

5. The process of dissociation is well demonstrated in the upper extremities as the infant progresses from gross to fine motor control. At first, motion is directed from the shoulder for swiping and batting. Later, the limb can accommodate innumerable positions of the joints for reach and manipulation. The following points should be considered in planning intervention to dissociate arm movement:

   a. The infant initially reaches with both hands (bilateral reach) before a unilateral reach is demonstrated. Early reach patterns of the young infant are more controlled in a supine-lying than in a sitting position. As the child gets older, reaching across the midline of the body reinforces an integrated body scheme.

   b. Toys should be positioned to encourage the development of rotation in the upper limbs. A primitive reach is internally rotated at the shoulder and pronated in the forearm. Consequently, the arm approaches the toy from above in a downward direction (a "top-level" reach). Only later with the emergence of external rotation and supination can the arm approach the object from the side.

      Supination is often coordinated during hand-to-mouth play. The infant first mouths the dorsum (back) of the hand since the forearm remains pronated. Over time, supination positions the hand for sucking the fingers and eventually the thumb. Mouthing objects and finger feeding provide opportunities to practice controlled supination. In similar fashion, the infant first exhibits vertical banging of the arms before acquiring the external rotation and supination required for horizontal clapping.

   c. Learning to grade motion at the elbow is often achieved in prone lying as the infant pushes up on extended arms and bounces. The degree of elbow extension when reaching appears related to the infant's ability to assume and maintain this gross motor position. Midrange control of the elbow is also fostered by playing with rattles, mobiles, pull toys, and popbeads.

   d. The development of isolated wrist movement facilitates the appearance of skilled prehension. In the beginning, the infant will tend to grasp objects with the wrist flexed. The goal is to achieve a stable wrist in slight extension during manipulative play. Coordination of wrist motion is practiced when the infant rocks in antigravity positions while bearing weight on the hands or when he or she pivots on the abdomen in a circle. Later activities—those requiring grasp, release, dumping, pouring, and hammering—refine this control. As previously discussed, grading the work surface can also be used to elicit gradation of wrist extension in busy box–type activities.

e. Opposition of the thumb is the key to acquiring fine prehensile patterns. It allows the thumb to approximate the ends of the index and middle fingers in a two- or three-point pinch. The digits are then positioned for the discrete manipulation of objects.

The type of grasp prehension used by the child depends in large measure on the size and position of the object to be handled. For example, a child will tend to use a radial-digital grasp to pick up a 1-inch block but a neat pincer (fingertip) grasp to retrieve a small pellet. The hand accommodates to the dimensions of the object. Consequently, the clinician should analyze which grasp and prehensile patterns can be elicited by objects of varying sizes and shapes. Fine motor activities are sequenced to expand the repertoire of grasp, release, and manipulative skills (e.g., tearing and crumpling paper, playing with a busy box or pegboard, transferring objects in and out of containers).

Promoting Fine Motor Control

There are numerous activities that can be employed to promote fine motor control in the child with myelomeningocele.

Emptying and Filling Activities Developmentally, a child learns to empty a container before filling it and does so with solids before liquids. In the beginning, the child often engages in these take-out and put-in activities with pegs, blocks, or beads and a bucket. Pots, pans, and utensils of different sizes are used in play with sand or water. A turkey baster is particularly effective for strengthening the hands during water play. Pouring and filling skills can also be practiced using uncooked kidney beans, a scoop, and a container.

Paper Tearing and Crumpling Depending on the child's level of functioning, the resistance of the paper can be graded from light news print to heavy construction paper. In teaching paper tearing, the adult first initiates the tear and holds one side of the paper while the child tears it from the other end. The next step is for the child to hold the paper with two hands and tear it apart after the adult has started the tear. Finally, the child can handle the complete task independently. After tearing, the paper can be crumpled with both hands and glued to another sheet for a collage. Or it can be rolled into little balls and flicked with the fingers across the table. In this activity, isolated finger extension is encouraged.

Fingerpainting The activity of fingerpainting stimulates gross arm movements in unilateral and bilateral patterns as well as dissociation of the fingers. Yogurt or pudding are excellent media for toddlers who tend to bring hands to the mouth. Preschool children can use regular fingerpaints, shaving cream, or Crazy Foam. The work surface can be adjusted to a horizontal, inclined, or vertical plane. Playing on a large mirror adds special interest to the task.

Clay Activities Clay, putty, or Play-Doh provides an opportunity to develop strength and coordination in the upper extremities. Since these media are free form, they foster imaginative play and guarantee success. The activity can be graded by rolling the clay into long cylinders ("hot dogs") with one or both hands pressed against the work surface. Rolling the clay into round balls requires more coordination, particularly if each hand rolls a separate ball on the table. Of greater difficulty is the use of reciprocal movements of the hands together in the air to make clay balls. Strengthening is enhanced by squeezing the clay, pushing fingers through the medium to make a tunnel, or molding animals or sculptures.

Finger Games Books are commercially available describing finger games of varying levels of complexity. These action songs foster motor planning, gestural imitation, language, and social interaction. Gross arm movements are practiced in such games as "Pat-a-Cake" and "Little Rabbit in the Wood"; finger movements are required in "Itsy Bitsy Spider." For the older child, shadow figures can be made with the fingers.

Bead Stringing The child can learn the concepts required for bead stringing by the use of a large rubberized board with holes. At first, the adult places the string in a hole, and the child pulls it through from the other side. In the next step, the child learns to place the string in a hole with the adult pulling it through. Finally, the child can sequence both steps—push in and pull out—to execute the task independently.

After use of the board, large beads are introduced following the same instructional procedure. With the adult holding the bead, the child can learn the activity using one hand before graduating to a bilateral approach (i.e., use of two hands).

Cutting with Scissors Depending on the child's level of functioning, three different types of scissors can be used. "E-Z grip" scissors require only a squeezing motion in order to cut. The child holds the scissors with a gross grasp. Four-hole training scissors enable the adult to assist the child in hand-over-hand fashion. The regular two-hole scissors are available with either a regular blunt or sharp cutting edge and for right- or left-handed use.

This task can also be graded by varying the resistance of the paper and the degree of assistance in holding the paper. The child first learns to produce simple snipping motions and cuts very short strips. Later, continuous motion is required for cutting straight lines across a page and then for cutting shapes.

Pencil or Crayon Use Two factors are initially considered in planning a program to achieve manipulation of a crayon or pencil with a static tripod grasp. First, the child should be sufficiently familiar with crayons to be interested in using them appropriately. For example, the child is able to scribble on paper and demonstrates some purposeful intent to make strokes for symbolic representation. Second, the child should demonstrate a lateral prehension or a neat pincer grasp when holding objects before a pencil grasp can be expected. Thus, activities that will refine the manipulation of small objects should be introduced prior to a program geared toward developing a static or dynamic tripod grasp. For the preschool-age child, a mature pincer grasp with objects is encouraged in such activities as building with small Lego pieces, peeling and pasting stickers, pinching clothespins, and stringing small (½-inch) beads.

Often, it is helpful to provide the child with additional sensory feedback when a mature grasp of the pencil or crayon is introduced. Scribbling on sandpaper, corrugated paper, or paper taped over an embossed and textured board provides the child with added kinesthetic feedback to reinforce the grasp pattern. Likewise, crayons or pencils can be graded in size from wide to narrow as the child's skill progresses. Compensatory techniques can also be explored if the child is unable to grasp adequately due to motor incoordination or abnormal muscle tone. These alternatives include the use of a plastic triangle-shaped holder (grip) inserted over a pencil, or pencils with molded shafts that facilitate proper finger placement when held.

Prewriting Activities Prewriting skills include those activities that most children accomplish with a crayon or pencil prior to writing. They emerge in the toddler years when the child begins to imitate vertical and horizonal strokes. Imitating circles and crosses follows at approximately 3–4 years of age. Later, the child learns to imitate basic shapes, including squares and triangles. Whether learning to draw single lines or geometric shapes, a typical sequence of development is followed. The child first imitates the adult's action, then copies from a model, and finally initiates the drawing from memory.

To construct vertical lines, for example, the child imitates the movements of an adult drawing lines from top to bottom on a large piece of paper. Next, the child may learn to trace over lines. Finally, the child practices making vertical lines, with two dots used as starting and stopping points, as well as making vertical lines without a model. In the case of learning to draw geometric shapes, tracing sometimes precedes imitating and copying. Tracing is useful if the child has difficulty visualizing how to make the shape.

Prewriting skills are fostered by coloring and painting in progressively smaller boundaries, connecting dots with "roads" (dot-to-dot activities), playing chalkboard games, and tracing on top of masking tape designs. Educational materials and curricular programs are commercially available for use with preschool- and school-age children. However, it is important to consider carefully the child's developmental level prior to selecting a published training program. The majority of these prewriting programs are not recommended for children under 4–5 years of age.

◇ CHAPTER 7 ◇

Speech and Language

COMMUNICATION IS A COMPLICATED PROCESS OF MESSAGES GOING BETWEEN A sender and a recipient. Language is the code in which the messages are sent, through a system of signals that may take the form of gestures, signs, or words. A breakdown in communication results when the message either is not properly encoded (i.e., the language is not clearly formulated by the sender) or is not properly decoded (i.e., the language is not correctly interpreted by the receiver). This chapter discusses the kinds of problems that may occur in the acquisition of language by some children with spina bifida. In order to enhance understanding, it begins with a review of normal language development.

NORMAL LANGUAGE DEVELOPMENT

According to Bloom and Lahey (1978), language has three parts: 1) content (the meaning of the message), 2) form (the way in which sounds and words are connected), and 3) use (the purpose of the communication). In the utterance "Bert jump," two words, a noun and a verb (form), are used to talk about a person doing an action (content) for the purpose of reporting an ongoing event in play (use). The integration of these parts is critical to the understanding (receiving) and expression (sending) of messages.

Language learning begins in early infancy, long before the child utters a first word, and continues throughout the formative years. Infants and young children acquire language through interaction with their environment, which is experienced through the senses by touching, seeing, hearing, and smelling. Gradually, the information obtained through the senses is organized in increasingly sophisticated ways as the child learns to communicate with people about objects and events.

Developing Language Content

Prerequisite skills are developed by the infant that eventually lead to an ability to label objects, express what they do, and describe their characteristics. The following competencies are instrumental in the development of language content during infancy:

1. The ability to attend visually and auditorily to people and objects in the environment.
2. The knowledge that something exists when it is no longer in view. The infant may demonstrate this ability by crying when the caregiver disappears from sight or by searching for hidden objects.
3. The imitation of gestures. For example, the infant is able to imitate a movement associated with a familiar phrase, such as raising the hands when the adult exclaims "So big!"
4. The imitation of sounds. A child may imitate nonlinguistic sounds, such as "ah-ba," and later linguistic sounds, such as "bye-bye."
5. The manipulation of objects, using increasingly more complex strategies. A child initially employs simple actions such as mouthing or shaking a toy before progressing to more complex behaviors such as ring stacking.
6. The ability to solve simple problems. An infant may demonstrate this ability by crawling some distance to play with an object or by pulling a string to obtain a toy. There is a strong relationship between problem-solving skills and the symbolic use of language.

During the toddler stage of development, children typically become more mobile. They utilize movement—crawling, cruising, and walking—to explore the environment and to manipulate objects. They attempt to negotiate stairs, pull open drawers, or dump the garbage can, and they enjoy throwing objects and then retrieving them from under chairs or tables. Also specific to the toddler are increased self-initiated periods of symbolic play and an expanded ability to imitate novel sounds and words.

During the preschool years, the child acquires the following competencies relating to the content of language:

1. The ability to group objects according to their function (e.g., all things that are eaten), association (e.g., things that belong together such as hand and mitten), and common attributes (e.g., classifying by shape or color).
2. The ability to describe objects according to their qualities (e.g., "I want the big ball" or "I want the fast truck" or "The car has round wheels").
3. The ability to understand and describe spatial relations such as position (on/in), distance (near/far), and direction (to/from).
4. The ability to sequence pictures that tell a story or to discuss events that occurred in the course of the day. The child begins to evidence an understanding of time by using such words as "tomorrow" and "yesterday."

Developing Language Form

Skills relating to the form of language are those that help the child learn ways of putting sounds together to make a word, ways of putting words together to form an utterance, and ways of putting utterances together to achieve a complete message.

The development of sound production proceeds in a characteristic sequence. The infant initially produces differentiated cries to express such feelings as hunger or pain. Oral and nasal vowel-like cooing sounds are also often heard and are frequently produced with movement. By 4–5 months, the infant begins to babble and produces consonant-vowel combinations such as "da-da" or "ga-ga." At 7–9 months, the infant produces reduplicated babbling sequences, such as "ga-ga-ga," and attempts to imitate similar sound patterns produced by another.

By 1 year, the child is attempting some word approximations and is continuing to acquire a variety of new speech sounds. Sounds in differentiated intonation patterns and pitch inflections are produced in jargon sequences that sound like true conversational sentences. Also, the child's attempts at imitating new words become increasingly accurate. The use of single words is followed by simple two-word combinations, such as "Daddy push" or "my cookie."

During the preschool years, the child learns to form complete sentences, such as "Daddy push the ball" or "I eat a cookie." More complex utterances develop over time, such as "I will push the ball when I take it out of the box." The child also demonstrates increased knowledge of grammatical rules and can use pronouns, plurals, and verb tense (past and future forms).

Developing Language Use

Appropriate use of language involves the mastery of such conversational rules as turn taking between the speaker and listener, the use of nonverbal cues during communication, and the use of utterances for varied purposes.

Eye gaze between caregiver and infant is the earliest behavior considered to be "communicative" in nature. Eye gaze is followed by vocalization and smiling as means of responding to the caregiver's verbal and facial expressions. The infant's random vocalizations become reinforced when imitated by the caregiver, and the infant learns to initiate vocalization to gain attention. Reciprocal vocalization between caregiver and child then forms the basis of conversational interchange, with the infant imitating sounds and, later, words. At the same time, the infant becomes increasingly attentive to gestures performed by an adult. In the game of peek-a-boo, for example, this attentiveness begins with looking and laughing or vocalizing, and eventually leads to imitation of the adult's gestures by the infant. Other examples of early gestural communicative games are "So Big" and "Pat-a-Cake."

Pointing, giving, and showing are early gestures to call attention to an interesting object or to get the adult to do something. During the toddler stage, these gestures, in combination with eye gaze and vocalizing, are major conversational devices. Vocal skills are characterized by the use of jargon (sound sequences that are unintelligible but sound like sentences), word approximation, and imitation of adult words and phrases. When pretending to talk on a toy telephone, for example, the toddler may produce jargon-like utterances that sound like one side of a typical phone conversation. This ability demonstrates knowledge of verbal turn-taking skills that the young child acquires for later use in formal conversation.

As the child's expressive vocabulary grows, words are used for many purposes or functions: to label ("cup"), to make a request ("want cookie"), and to report detail ("big cookie"). Later, in the preschool years, the child uses language for more abstract functions such as reasoning about causal relationships ("He's crying because his finger hurts"), predicting events or consequences ("She will get mad because I broke it"), and requesting information ("Why did the man get mad?").

PROBLEMS IN SPEECH AND LANGUAGE DEVELOPMENT

It is important to emphasize that many children with spina bifida develop normal speech and language abilities. However, some children with myelomeningocele and hydrocephalus are prone to deficits in language functioning that appear related to increased distractibility and limitations in selective attention (Horn et al., 1985). Various factors may contribute to the inability of a child with myelomeningocele to develop speech and language normally, including:

1. Poor attending behaviors
2. Hypersensitivity to auditory, tactile, and visual stimuli
3. Difficulties in visual-motor coordination, spatial orientation, and figure-ground perception
4. Limitations in gross and fine motor skills
5. Long illnesses or hospitalizations
6. Cognitive impairment

Research has tended to focus on the language problems of school-age children with spina bifida, rather than on infants and toddlers. But clinical experience reveals difficulties with prelinguistic play and interactional skills in some young children, as well as delays in the production of first words. More research is needed to document the specific kinds of problems displayed early in life.

Prelinguistic Play and Interaction

The infant with myelomeningocele usually displays deficiencies in gross motor skills and is therefore limited in the ability to move and to explore the environment independently. Also, poor development of manipulative skills may hamper the child's ability to explore toys in a variety of action schemes. In addition, hospitalization or orthopaedic surgery or shunt revisions may decrease the child's opportunity for exploratory learning. Interaction with people may also be limited to a few family members. As a result, delays are sometimes noted in the ability to play with others, in the development of gestural and vocal/verbal imitation, and in early social responses. In many cases, however, vocalization, vocal imitation, and social responsiveness are areas of strength in infants with spina bifida. Because they lack movement, social responses and vocalization with others may be the major means for these infants to reach out and communicate with their environment.

First Words

Distractibility and perceptual problems may interfere with the child's ability to understand and use words. As a result, the toddler may exhibit a delay in the acquisition of a receptive and expressive vocabulary. If the child with myelomeningocele and hydrocephalus is easily distracted or unable to screen out unimportant visual or auditory stimuli, difficulty may arise in distinguishing important perceptual features of objects (e.g., size, shape, texture) and in developing the meaning of words to describe them (e.g., attributes such as round or smooth). Delays may also occur in the comprehension and use of early words describing such characteristics as spatial location (in, on, under), comparative size (big, bigger), or time (morning, night, yesterday).

Conversation

A semantic-pragmatic problem that may be exhibited once the child has acquired verbal skills has been labeled the "cocktail party syndrome." This dysfunction refers to a good ability to use language forms (sentences and grammatical structure) but difficulty with the content (meaning) and use (functions and purpose) of language (Rahlson, 1983). The likelihood of children displaying hyperverbal behavior increases when there is below average intelligence or in the presence of hydrocephalus with or without shunts.

Since the emergence of language in these children is often viewed very positively, as offsetting or even compensating for deficits in motor abilities, unrelated responses may be fostered and maintained by adults. However, irrelevant verbalization appears to decrease with age, possibly as a result of the structure provided in the classroom and the language demands of teachers and peers (Tew, 1979).

The following features are characteristic of the cocktail party syndrome:

1. Difficulty paying attention to language when there is competing background noise (e.g., traffic, air conditioning, other children playing)
2. Continuous talking
3. Ability to use words in conversation but poor comprehension of their meaning
4. Precocious use of a sophisticated, adultlike vocabulary
5. Inability to establish or maintain a topic in conversation

6. Excessive use of social phrases such as "Oh, come on" or social routines such as greetings (e.g., continually saying "Hi")
7. Responses that are social or personal in nature rather than related to the topic
8. Inappropriate use of words due to lack of comprehension
9. Difficulty using language to reason
10. Difficulty answering "wh" questions (i.e., who, what, where, when, why)
11. Difficulty terminating or changing topics within a conversation
12. Difficulty following lengthy directions
13. Difficulty comprehending stories and answering questions related to details, main ideas, and the sequence of events

BASES FOR INTERVENTION

Play and Cognitive Development in Infants and Toddlers

A child's ability to play with objects and explore the environment contributes to the development of language. The Uzgiris-Hunt Ordinal Scales of Psychological Development, based on Piaget's description of the sensorimotor period of development, assess cognitive skills during the first 2 years of life. These skills contribute in varying degrees to the acquisition of language. Since the scales are a useful developmental frame of reference for practitioners, the discussion that follows emphasizes competencies described by Uzgiris and Hunt (1975). Sample activities and strategies for intervention are provided in each area. (Dunst, 1981, is another useful reference for assessing and planning prelinguistic intervention.)

Visual Pursuit and the Permanence of Objects   Object permanence is the understanding that an object continues to exist even though it is out of view. At approximately 4–6 months of age, a child will visually search for an object at the point of disappearance. The infant visually follows an object falling from sight, particularly if he or she was previously handling it. Likewise, the infant follows the caregiver's movements about the room and will gaze at the spot where the adult just left the room. Later, the infant will search for an object partially hidden by a cloth or screen. By 8 months, the child will uncover a toy totally hidden under a cloth after observing the adult hide it. Over time this skill develops, so that the child can locate an object after it has been hidden under a series of screens. This cognitive awareness of the permanent existence of objects is important because it may contribute to the child's growing ability to talk about objects that are not in the perceptual field (Bloom & Lahey, 1978).

Intervention   To enhance this skill, the clinician first begins with tasks that promote visual fixation and tracking. (Chapter 6 discusses numerous strategies to promote these visual abilities.) Next, the practitioner can play modified hide-and-seek games with the infant. Visually stimulating objects are partially hidden within reach of the child in order to elicit an active retrieval. Gradually, the complexity of the activity is increased by following the previously mentioned developmental sequence. In the beginning, it is important to allow the infant to observe the hiding of the object as a cue to solicit searching.

Purposeful Problem Solving Purposeful problem solving is involved when a child begins to develop simple ways to achieve a desired end. For example, the young infant will use visually directed reaching to explore an attractive mobile or toy placed in the crib. When multiple objects are involved, a child at the age of 7 months will drop one or more objects held in the hands to obtain a newly presented object. Means-ends skill is a strong predictor for the development of language (Bates, Benigni, Bretherton, Camaioni, & Volterra, 1979).

Intervention Having the child pull a string to obtain a toy or to activate it is one play activity that develops means-ends or problem-solving abilities. Oscar the Grouch in a garbage can or toy dogs that make noises when moved are inviting pull toys. The task is made easier by shortening the string or tying a plastic ring to the end of it. The child can also learn to retrieve toys that are hung from the high chair on lengths of yarn. Purposeful problem solving is further facilitated by having the infant learn to obtain an object out of immediate reach by pulling a towel on which the object rests. The development of gross motor skills, such as crawling, pulling to stand, or walking, are other means for obtaining desired ends such as objects that the caregiver has deliberately placed out of reach.

Causality Cause-and-effect relationships develop as an infant begins to anticipate events. The child acquires strategies for stimulating objects or people to create interesting sights and sounds. For example, an infant may display general body movements such as leg kicking or arm waving to elicit a repeat performance of the adult's caresses and kisses. Infants as early as 3 months will repeat an arm movement to keep a toy activated.

Intervention It is important for adults to be sensitive to the infant's signals that communicate a wish for an action to be repeated. Cause-effect behaviors can be developed through many of the common activities of daily living, such as flipping on light switches, opening and closing drawers, and turning knobs.

Spatial Relationships The term "spatial relationships" refers to the infant's ability to appreciate the orientation of objects and sounds in space, and their relation to the self and to each other. A young infant develops the ability to look for and localize sound. For example, the infant learns to locate the caregiver's voice through visual gaze when the adult is in close proximity and then at greater distances across the room.

Intervention Brightly colored, noise-making toys can be used to facilitate visual and auditory attention to the stimuli. The young infant can follow the course of the object as the adult moves it in horizonal and vertical directions. As the infant begins to reach for objects and hold them, a variety of rattles and toys should be made available. The infant is encouraged to turn objects around to look at all sides. A toy with a mirror on one side stimulates the child to turn it over for exploration. Further activities to foster spatial relations include placing objects in containers and dumping out the contents, building towers with blocks, and rolling toys down various inclines.

With increased mobility in the environment, awareness of the body in space is enhanced through having the child move around and between furniture. Placing obstacles in the child's way encourages the solving of spatial problems—the infant learns to take a detour around the obstacles to obtain a desired object. (Chapter 6 provides additional suggestions for enhancing spatial relationships.)

Play Schemes with Objects   The cognitive area of play schemes with objects refers to an infant's ability to initiate a variety of play actions with toys. As infants develop, their repertoire of play actions enlarges. Initial play schemes include holding, mouthing, and looking at toys. Eventually, the infant learns to shake, wave, and bang the toys. Complex motor actions emerge over time as the child learns more diverse strategies for manual play such as behaviors involving letting go, throwing, and combining objects in play.

Intervention   Early action schemes can be facilitated when the child with spina bifida is securely positioned. Rattles, spoons, and toys that produce auditory feedback encourage banging and hitting. Activities that promote more complex motor actions include pulling tissues from a box, crumbling and ripping paper, sliding or pushing cars on sand, or moving boats in water. The ability to combine objects in play is enhanced through pulling apart or putting together pop beads, putting objects into containers and taking them out again, stacking blocks, and putting rings on a ring stack.

Symbolic Play   The development of symbolic play is a higher-level play skill that is an important prerequisite for language. Through activities involving symbolic play, the child demonstrates knowledge of the use of objects and imitates the previously observed actions of adults. Children first learn to carry out the pretend actions on themselves; later, they are able to pretend with a doll or an adult. The next step is to model pretend actions in sequence (e.g., pouring juice, then drinking). Pretend play becomes a major focus of toddler activity. A significant change that occurs between 18 and 24 months is that the child is able to use one object to represent or signify another. For example, a block can be used as a pretend cookie.

Actions or gestures that a child performs during symbolic play correlate with the attainment of early words (Bates et al., 1979). For example, a child who pretends to eat or drink may say "Juice, cookie, all-gone." Westby (1980) has suggested that the ability to combine words emerges at the same time a child combines gestures (e.g., pretends to stir with a spoon and then eat) or performs several actions on numerous people or objects.

Intervention Early symbolic play can be encouraged by playing with spoons, cups, and plates to model stirring, dishing out food, drinking, eating, or blowing on hot food. Washing and drying the dishes can also be a part of the play sequence.

Since the child with myelomeningocele may have limited gross motor ability to explore and interact with the broader environment, symbolic play activities using dolls or miniature toy people to perform actions is particularly helpful for promoting learning and language development. Many toys are available that can be employed for symbolic play, such as fire houses, barns, gas stations, and school houses—all with appropriate people and vehicles. Puppets, Sesame Street characters, and stuffed animals can also stimulate play episodes. The child's play sequences can be fostered by initially imitating the child's actions and then modeling novel activities or routines for the child to imitate.

Interactive and Communicative Development in Infants and Toddlers

Infants acquire the skills necessary for the development of language through interaction with their caregivers. These early interactional behaviors expand from gazing, smiling, and vocalizing to the use of gestures and imitation.

The earliest "communicative" interaction occurs between the infant and caregiver during feeding and face-to-face exchange. Field (1978) has suggested that such interaction is characterized by rhythm patterns, changing response repertoires, and the level of responsiveness of both caregiver and the infant. The rhythm patterns correspond with the infant's alert periods. Over time, the infant is able to remain alert for longer periods, and the adult learns to identify and control these periods for interaction. The term "response repertoires" refers to the different kinds of responses that a caregiver and infant display when interacting, such as facial expressions, gazing, and the infant's body movements. Adults often imitate a baby's responses, which in turn seems to elicit the infant's attention and desire to respond. The infant soon learns that initiation of a behavior by one evokes responses by the other. For example, gurgles by the infant stimulate the adult to gurgle or smile back. The infant also learns to initiate behaviors—laughing, smiling, crying, and vocalizing—to gain the adult's attention. Early development of interaction between caregiver and infant is the foundation for the development of communication.

It is important, therefore, that parents have the opportunity to spend time with their infant from the beginning, even when the newborn is hospitalized for required medical care. Depending on the medical status, parents may be able to hold, feed, and interact with the child, particularly during alert periods. As the infant stabilizes medically, the parents learn to recognize the child's response repertoire. Play is encouraged through making a variety of vocal noises, imitating the baby's behaviors, and gentle stroking. The parents may initially require emotional support in order to develop feelings of attachment to their baby and to become comfortable in handling the young infant.

Vocal Imitation   Initially, infants imitate sounds of the adult that are already in their repertoire. By approximately 12 months of age, they learn to imitate novel sounds.

Vocal imitation is an important factor for the development of an expressive vocabulary. Likewise, the turn taking that is involved in imitative games fosters knowledge of conversational skills. Children continue to imitate words and phrases even when they have developed an expressive vocabulary that they are using to communicate. From 18 to approximately 24 months, the child will imitate novel words and complex verbalizations such as phrases or sentences. Even though these expressions may not be meaningful to the child or may merely be deferred imitation (i.e., imitating from memory), the act of imitation assists the child in the acquisition of an expressive vocabulary.

Intervention   Excellent times for vocalization to take place between the child and caregiver are during feeding and diaper changes, since physical proximity to adults appears to be a crucial stimulus for increasing vocalizations by the infant. For imitation to develop, the infant and the adult must have learned to engage in reciprocal vocalizations. That is, they must have learned to play the game in which one will coo or babble to elicit the other's vocal responses. At first, the caregiver should merely imitate the sounds that are made by the child, since the infant will most readily imitate sounds that he or she can already produce. The next step is to encourage the child to imitate novel sounds that are similar to the ones the infant can produce (e.g., if the infant can say "ba," the adult can attempt to elicit imitation of "da"). Attempts to approximate novel sounds should be reinforced.

Early sounds and words can be naturally modeled in the context of play or routine caregiving activities so as to promote understanding of the words. For example, the caregiver might ask if the infant wants to "go bye-bye." An early response would be a contingent, nonspecific vocalization ("ah"); at a later stage, the infant might respond "ba-ba"; and later yet, the infant will be able to imitate "bye-bye" accurately. All along, the simultaneous physical action of leaving one place and going to another reinforces that "bye-bye" means going away.

Gestural Imitation   Imitation of gestures proceeds along the same course as vocal imitation—from imitating the familiar to imitating the novel. Infants initially produce random movements in response to an adult's movements (e.g., banging the hands on the table in response to the adult shaking a rattle). Between 4 and 8 months, children will imitate simple gestures in their repertoire that are visible to themselves.

Intervention　Gestures to model for imitation include clapping hands for "Pat-a-Cake," arms up for "So Big," opening and closing the hands, or other actions that accompany simple songs. Gestural imitation can progress, between 8 and 12 months, to novel movements that comprise familiar actions (e.g., clapping the hands on the knees instead of together). The pairing of vocalization and gestures can be used to develop imitative skills. For example, patting one's nose can be paired with the vocalization "beep-beep." Simple songs such as "The Itsy Bitsy Spider" can be used to develop gestural and vocal imitations. Children's records that elicit gestures are also good facilitators of imitative skills. By 12–18 months, children can be encouraged to imitate complex, novel actions.

Nonverbal Communication　The use of expressive gestures such as pointing, giving, and showing seems to be related to the development of language (Bates et al., 1979). These gestural schemes appear at approximately 9–12 months of age and continue to be displayed in conjunction with the child's verbal efforts to communicate. Young children with myelomeningocele frequently use these nonverbal communicative behaviors, especially pointing and showing, to elicit an adult's attention or help. These behaviors are particularly useful for those children who have a limited ability to move through the environment to interact with objects and people.

For the child with spina bifida who appears to be delayed in producing words, introducing nonverbal communicative behaviors may be a facilitative technique—that is, it may help to promote language. It is important to note that gestural skills are influenced by the child's ability to maintain a sitting posture with the arms free for movement. When necessary, therefore, special seating should be provided to ensure adequate sitting balance.

Pointing　Pointing is employed to call an adult's attention to objects or to request specific objects or actions. Pointing can be facilitated through modeling by the adult in specific situations in which the adult knows the child wants a particular object such as a bottle, cookie, or favorite toy.

Giving　Giving behaviors are exhibited when the child hands an object to an adult. This action can take place for several reasons. The child may be asking the adult to perform an action on the toy that the child cannot do independently (e.g., activating a wind-up toy); or the child may be initiating interaction by giving the toy (e.g., "Play with me"); or the child may simply wish to share the object with another.

Gestural and verbal cues such as an outstretched hand and saying "Give it to me" are facilitators of giving behaviors. Also, by structuring the situation in such a way that the adult must activate or retrieve a toy in order for the child to be able to play with it, the adult can motivate the child to use this mode of nonverbal communication.

Showing　Showing objects is also a behavior used initially to gain an adult's attention. The child may use the eyes—gazing alternately at the adult and at the object—to share interest or excitement in the object. The child may also hand new or interesting toys to the adult to initiate interaction.

Showing behaviors usually occur when something unexpected or novel occurs. New toys can be presented to the child, and the adult can say "What do you have? Show me." When the child looks at the object and then the adult, or picks up the object and gazes at the adult, positive reinforcement by the adult should occur such as smiling or nodding the head. The practitioner can also model showing behaviors to the child as they both share the excitement of the new toy or the unexpected event.

Early Words Prelinguistic play activities are important to develop a child's knowledge of objects, actions, and their relationship that serves as the basis for learning early words. Imitative vocal and gestural skills are just as critical for the development of future conversational abilities. Thus, for any young child experiencing language delay, prelinguistic play and interactive skills are goals of intervention previous to the introduction of early words.

Intentional vocal communication (sounds or sound combinations) can occur at 9–12 months of age, which correlates with cognitive levels of Late 4 or Early 5 on the Uzgiris-Hunt scales (Miller, 1980). By approximately 18 months of age, children use words to communicate about the here and now and to comment on their own actions. According to Bloom and Lahey (1978), the content of their language includes the following types of meaning: existence (naming objects), nonexistence (no, all gone, no more), recurrence (more, again), rejection (no), attribution (big/little, good/bad), possession (mine, Mommy), action (go, eat, come), and location (in, on). Another system of classifying early words (Dore, 1975) identifies nine ways the child can use language: labeling, repeating, answering, requesting actions, requesting answers, calling, greeting, protesting, and practicing.

Intervention Imaginative play situations can be used to increase a child's understanding of the types of meaning in the content of language. This expanded awareness fosters the development of specific words. For example, play with a pitcher and cup can be used to facilitate the understanding of the concept of "recurrence." The adult pretends to refill the cup repeatedly in order for the child to receive more juice to drink imaginatively. The vocabulary word "more" is verbally modeled during the activity. Thus, the child is given a specific context for learning the word "more." Over time, the child may generalize the learning to ask the mother for "more" juice at home.

Therapeutic and educational activities to encourage the development of early words should take place in a quiet setting with minimal auditory or visual distractions. Poor attending behaviors, hypersensitivity to auditory, tactile, or visual stimuli, and perceptual difficulties are factors that may hamper the child's ability to develop speech and language normally. Simple manipulative activities with few materials presented should be used to focus the child on the intent of the activity (e.g., just two cups and one teapot, rather than the entire set, can be used when working on the word "more"). The use of pictures during intervention should be considered carefully based on the abilities of the child. Some children are not able to derive meaning from pictures.

Communicative Skills in the Preschool Child

The focus of intervention for preschool children with spina bifida varies according to individual needs and capabilities. Some children may have age-appropriate or superior language skills. Others may display mild language problems that are manifested in impaired auditory comprehension or difficulties in reasoning. Yet other children may have moderate to severe language disorders in association with attention, perceptual, or cognitive deficits.

The attainment of adequate speech and language in the preschool years is an important prerequisite for academic functioning in the primary years in school. Such skills as reading comprehension and the understanding of mathematical concepts are dependent on a language base. The ability to use language conversationally with peers is also vital to the acquisition of social and emotional skills.

As discussed earlier in this chapter, some children with myelomeningocele, particularly when associated with hydrocephalus, may display problems in the area of language content (i.e., poor comprehension or use of words to describe attributes such as shape, texture, or location). The other major area of difficulty is the occurrence of hyperverbal behavior or what has been called the "cocktail party syndrome." The following discussion therefore highlights intervention in these two areas.

Enhancing Language Content   The development of language content is closely related to the cognitive and perceptual experiences that accompany the appropriately modeled language. The goal of intervention is to help the child make associations between objects, between events, and among objects and events collectively. The child must also learn to formulate mental representations of himself or herself and of objects and events in the environment. These mental representations are the basis for meaning expressed linguistically. By participating in concrete activities, the child can learn to use language to express the meaning of events, to reason about them, and to talk about them in the present, past, and future tenses.

Because of poor gross and fine motor skills or prolonged hospitalization, some children with myelomeningocele may not have experienced a diversity of sensorimotor activities. Moreover, due to perceptual or attention deficits, they may have difficulty recognizing significant aspects or features of an activity. Intervention should provide a variety of activities paired with verbal expression of the significant aspect or event that the child should focus on. For example, to focus on the attribute of size, two cars may be offered for play, with one significantly larger than the other; verbal modeling would then focus on size ("The *big* car goes fast").

Many assessment tools are available for determining abilities in language content. However, most formal assessment instruments are picture-based, which may present difficulties for some children. Concrete activities involving real objects may have to be used instead. For example, when assessing knowledge of the concept "size," rather than presenting a picture of a big and little car, two toy cars should be presented with the verbal cue "Find the *big* car." In addition to the variety of assessment tools, there are curricula available that suggest goals and strategies for intervention.

The Cognitively Oriented Curriculum by Weikart (1971) and his associates, divides areas of language content into specific categories and presents intervention activities for each content area. In each case, the motor component of an activity is paired with a verbal aspect. For example, to teach classification one would present for manipulative play objects that differ in some respect, while using the words "same" and "not the same," as appropriate.

The content areas described by Weikart are classification, seriation, spatial relations, and temporal relations. In Table 7.1, activities are suggested for the first of these four areas, classification. For activities in the other content areas, the reader is referred to Weikart (1971).

The sample activities in the table can be used to develop the child's ability to use words to talk specifically about how objects are classified. The professional should be certain that the child is truly comprehending specific words and concepts by presenting them in a variety of play situations. The child may be using an adultlike vocabulary in conversation yet may be lacking a true understanding of the meaning of the words.

Enhancing Language Use and Conversation   During the preschool years, children become more sophisticated in their ability to use language. They are no longer primarily expressing wants and needs or describing objects and actions in the present. They begin to talk about events and objects not present in the immediate situation and display a variety of conversational skills. For example, over time the use of language to imitate, ask a question, or describe actions decreases in frequency. During this preoperational period of cognitive development, children also learn to continue the topic of an adult's conversation. The ability to add new information to a conversation begins to emerge at approximately 3 years of age (Bloom, Rocissano, & Hood, 1976).

Since some children with myelomeningocele are known to have particular difficulty in conversational situations, it is important for the clinician to analyze how a child uses language to interact with others. There are many different ways to analyze how language is used and how a speaker's utterance relates to a previous utterance. A review of pragmatic taxonomies has been provided in a text by Miller (1980). Dore (1978) has reported a method of organizing the

Table 7.1. Suggested activities in the content area of classification

I. Relational: Grouping items on the basis of common function and on the basis of association
  A. Have the children group together objects that have the same function; for example, things for eating (cup, spoon, plate) and things for wearing (shoes, socks, pants).
  B. Have the children match objects that are used for the same function but look different; for example, two different shoes, or a cup and a glass.
  C. Have the children match pictures of articles of clothing with pictures of corresponding body parts.
  D. Show pictures of objects and have the children act out the appropriate action; for example, show a picture of a broom and have the children sweep the floor with a pretend broom.

II. Descriptive: Grouping items on the basis of common attributes
  A. Have the children sort blocks or beads of different sizes, placing big ones in one group and little ones in the other.
  B. Have the children match objects that are the same shape.
  C. Have the children group pictures of big and little objects.
  D. Have the children sort objects or pictures of objects that are of different shape, color, and size.

III. Generic: Grouping items on the basis of general classes or categories
  A. Have the children sort objects according to category; for example, clothing, furniture, food.
  B. Have the children make a "category book" by pasting pictures that are "the same" into a booklet.
  C. Play category games, such as Lotto, in which the children have to match pictures that belong to the same category.
  D. Present four pictures with one that does not belong in the same category as the other three. Have the children pick it out and tell why it does not belong.

Source: Adapted from Weikart (1971).

conversational behaviors of preschool children into eight categories: requests, responses, descriptions, statements, acknowledgments, organizational devices (e.g., boundary markers such as "hi," "bye," or "okay," or politeness markers such as "thanks," or "sorry"), performatives (e.g. protests, jokes, or teasing), and miscellaneous.

Analyzing a child's conversational language helps to reveal incorrect patterns of language use. For example, the child may only respond to requests but not initiate them. When asked questions about past events, difficulty may be displayed in describing specific people, actions, or details. The child may have problems responding to questions about the who, what, where, when, and why of present or past events. Or the child may use organizational devices excessively because of an inability to interact fluently with another. The practitioner should identify specific patterns in language use and calculate their frequency of occurrence. If the child overuses organizational devices, the adult can direct comments to a relevant activity. If the child displays infrequent use of requesting behaviors, then developing requesting would be a goal of intervention.

Lucas (1980) has provided a comprehensive discussion of problems in language content and language use. She believes that children who are unable to maintain good eye contact—which is sometimes the case in children with spina bifida—often have problems in understanding the main topic of a conversation and in terminating a conversation. They also tend to resort to echolalia (repeating the words of another speaker).

Topic Maintenance Difficulty in maintaining the topic of a conversation may be due to an inability to understand or focus on the main idea of another's speech. Children who display this problem are described as having fluent speech but poor understanding; they continue to talk in situations where they do not understand the content of the conversation.

The adult should introduce a topic that is familiar to both participants either through a shared past experience or an event in the present context. The topic should be of interest to the child and at an appropriate level of comprehension. Rather than being allowed to dominate a conversation, the child must be provided with activities that give practice in following the intent or topic of another individual's conversation. It may be necessary to stop during an activity and ask the child to repeat what the adult just said. Pictures of objects or actions can be presented when important or main ideas are being discussed. The pictures provide cues for the child in order to focus on significant conversational points.

Role playing can provide an appropriate context for modeling responses for the child, with a third person demonstrating the appropriate utterance. Depending on the developmental level of the child, pictures can also be used. The adult should have the child pretend to be the person in the situation depicted by the picture, and should encourage him or her to make utterances appropriate for that role.

Topic Closure The child who is too talkative may be having difficulty terminating the discussion of a topic. To overcome this problem, the child needs to learn: 1) to be aware of linguistic markers, 2) to recognize the boundaries of a topic, and 3) to understand the content of what has been said.

Lucas (1980) has suggested the following approaches to promote topic closure:

1. The adult begins with narrow topics and questions about specific events (e.g., "What did you do during free play?").
2. The adult reiterates the child's answer so that the child hears what he or she said (e.g., "So, you played with the blocks and peg board").
3. The adult paces the dialogue by interrupting verbally if the child rambles in conversation. Brisk pacing helps to frame utterances and mark boundaries.
4. When answering a question, the adult replaces indefinite pronouns with the same words used in the question ("Yes, it is an alligator," rather than "Yes, it is").

A child with problems in topic closure may ramble and rephrase previous utterances. The child may provide new but irrelevant information that is merely tangential to the topic. According to Lucas (1980), two techniques are useful for correcting tangentiality: 1) avoiding tangential utterances by narrowing the topic and keeping the child on target with close-ended questions, and 2) redirecting the child so that the topic limits are known (e.g., it is appropriate for the adult to say directly to the child, "We are not talking about _____, we are talking about _____").

Using Language to Reason   A major objective in the preschool years is the development of language to the point where the child is able to use language for reasoning and solving problems. For example, the preschool child should be able to perform sequences of symbolic play, to understand his or her own actions as separate and influencing those of another, and to understand how events are causally related.

Some children with spina bifida who are conversationally skillful may display problems with these types of higher-level language uses. It may be necessary, for instance, to design activities to develop predicting behaviors. Situations such as cooking can be structured to focus on prediction ("What will happen if we forget to put in the sugar?" or "What should we do after we mix the batter?"). Gradually, the context for predicting behaviors can progress from concrete situations to pictures and stories.

One orientation to language use stresses the role of discourse between the child and teacher in the preschool classroom (Blank, Rose, & Berlin, 1978). Four levels of complexity in the discourse between teacher and child have been suggested:

1. *Matching perception* involves reporting and responding to salient information. A task on this level entails, for example, naming objects.
2. *Selective analysis of perception* involves the exchange of less salient information; for example, describing shape, size or texture.
3. *Reordering perception* requires using language to rearrange perceptual input; for example, identifying which item does not belong in an activity requiring categorization.
4. *Reasoning about perception,* the most difficult level, involves the use of language to make associations and integrate ideas and relationships.

Language for instruction should be at the level of discourse in which the child can participate. If a child can converse only at the first level (matching perception), then the majority of questions should emphasize naming objects or pictures. The level of difficulty is increased slowly over time. A distractible child may find group activities particularly demanding, and attention deficits may interfere with learning language in these situations.

Practitioners need to know the strengths and weaknesses of the child in the use of language for reasoning. The child may display difficulty understanding

◇ CHAPTER 8 ◇

Activities of Daily Living

A MAJOR ACHIEVEMENT IN THE EARLY CHILDHOOD YEARS IS THE DEVELOPment of increasing independence in activities of daily living. The ability to take care of one's own needs in such self-care tasks as dressing, bathing, and eating contributes significantly to a sense of competence and self-esteem. The child with spina bifida requires guidance in the early years to acquire such independence. Physical limitations, learning difficulties, and possible overdependence on adults may interfere with mastery of the self-care skills.

This chapter focuses on the special needs of children with myelomeningocele in the following areas: dressing, bathing, bowel and bladder management, feeding and diet, and transfers. Practical suggestions are provided in each area for promoting the child's self-reliance.

DRESSING AND BRACING

Dressing

The development of dressing skills progresses in a predictable sequence during early childhood. It begins with the young child cooperating with the caregiver (e.g., positioning the arms for removal of a pullover garment) and attempting to remove socks and shoes. During the preschool years, the child eventually learns to put on clothes and gradually masters fasteners such as zippers, buttons, and buckles.

Dressing is a sophisticated perceptual-motor task requiring the integration of several subskills. The child must have an awareness of the relation of the parts of the body to each other and to the whole, and their position in space, in order to plan required movements. Postural control for balance must be combined with upper-extremity reach, grasp, and manipulation in order to accomplish such activities as putting on pants or shoes. Visual-spatial skills are necessary for learning to turn clothing right side out and positioning garments in the proper orientation for dressing. For example, awareness of right and left sides of the body in relation to clothing is essential for more difficult tasks such as donning a shirt that opens in front. Finally, mastery of dressing skills requires that one be able to sequence the various component steps of each task from start to finish in a systematic fashion.

Most children with spina bifida have the potential for independence in dressing, although the rate of acquisition of skills may be slower than is normally expected. Since dressing skills are complex, it is important that the young child be provided with the early preparatory experiences that foster later independence. Due to the child's physical limitations, independent or assisted dressing may take more time. Busy family schedules often make it easier for family members to dress and undress the child, particularly in the early morning. When this is the case, dressing skills can be practiced at bedtime and on weekends. Care should be taken that adults grade the assistance provided. A natural response is to do the activity for the child in order to save time and energy. Such a pattern, however, furthers dependence rather than facilitating independent behavior.

Several factors can interfere with the development of dressing skills in children with spina bifida. These factors include insufficient motor control, sensory deficits, and delays in developing manipulative and perceptual skills. Poor sitting balance is the most common motor problem interfering with performance in dressing. When one or both hands are required for support to maintain independent sitting, dressing is severely restricted. Providing external support for sitting, or selecting alternate positions, frequently makes the difference between dependence on caregivers and independent functioning. The following positions may be considered to assist the dressing task:

1. The child is held in sitting on the adult's lap so that the child's arms are free to practice pulling off shoes, socks, and pants from the lower portion of the legs.
2. The child can sit on the floor while dressing with the back against a wall or an item of furniture. A floor seat or triangle chair can be used if lateral support is also required.
3. When the child sits independently but requires the security of an external support, a low stool or chair can be positioned next to the child for use as needed.
4. Supine lying is frequently the position of choice for putting on or taking off pants.

Lack of muscle innervation and decreased sensation in the legs are other common factors that affect dressing. The child does not feel the position of the legs and feet when putting on clothes. Removal and replacement of shoes, socks, and pants become more difficult when active leg movements and sensation are absent. Nevertheless, independence in these tasks can generally be achieved with guidance. When sensation is absent in the feet, teaching the donning of shoes is indicated when the child has adequate judgment to position feet in shoes in such a way as to avoid injury to toes and circulatory problems. When movement of the legs is absent, the child is taught compensatory methods of dressing that rely on passively moving and positioning the legs for the activity.

In preparation for the reach and grasp patterns necessary for dressing, play activities that require similar arm movements and manipulative skills are incorporated into daily activities. For example, to prepare for overhead reach in pulling off a shirt, the infant is engaged in games such as "So Big" or play involving putting on and taking off hats. The toddler can be encouraged to reach for objects overhead, such as popping bubbles, or can be engaged in action songs that involve reaching up and behind the head.

The grasp patterns necessary for holding onto clothing and later manipulating buttons and zippers is encouraged by the child holding a pillow case or paper bag in one hand, and putting in and taking out objects with the other hand. Play with pegs, puzzles, and plastic chips reinforces the use of pinch patterns. Preparation for buttoning is emphasized by inserting large buttons or plastic chips into slots cut out in various positions in a plastic container.

For the young infant, dressing provides repeated opportunities to develop body awareness and later, recognition of body parts. Body exploration is encouraged with "Pat-a-Cake" games and assisted foot-to-foot and hands-to-knees/feet play. It is important to position the young child so that he or she can observe the dressing procedures. While it is easier for the adult to dress and undress a young child in the supine position on a bed or table, positioning the child in supported sitting on the adult's lap encourages visual attention and participation.

Dressing the older child in front of a mirror can be helpful in some cases. Verbal interaction with the child during dressing is important for learning body parts. For example, the adult can point out that socks go on the feet and arms go through the sleeves. Over time, the child will begin to recognize body parts and will associate them with clothing items.

In preparation for teaching specific dressing skills, it is helpful to analyze each task in order to delineate the steps required for completion. Initially, it may be easier for the child to accomplish only the last step of the activity; then, the last two steps. Gradually, the number of steps are increased until the dressing sequence is learned. This approach uses a "backward chaining" technique. In teaching the removal of pants, for example, the child is first expected only to pull the pants off the feet. Later, the pants are pulled down from the knees and yet later, from the thighs and hips.

Use of the "hand-over-hand" method in guiding the child's movements is a common teaching technique. The child's hands are positioned to grasp the clothing with the adult's hands on top. The adult provides the physical cuing to assist the child's action. The following dressing procedures are helpful to foster independence.

Donning and Doffing Pants in a Reclined Position   The child begins in sitting with the legs out straight. The pants are positioned at the feet, ready for the legs to be placed into the top opening. The child pulls the pants up to the thighs, using one arm to lift the leg if there is no active movement. At this point, the child who has some degree of hip extension and knee flexion lies on the back. By lifting the buttocks up in a "bridging" position, the child pulls the pants over the hips. The child who lacks hip extension can assume side lying and pull the pants over the top hip. Rolling onto the other side, the child completes the task by pulling the pants over the other hip. Frequently, it is easier to zip and fasten the pants while lying on the back. This procedure is reversed for removal of the garment.

Self-Diapering   If the child is incontinent, self-diapering is taught at an early age. It is realistic to expect a toddler to participate actively in the process. While most children accomplish diaper removal with ease, adult supervision is generally necessary for maintaining hygiene. Independent donning of diapers is easiest in supine lying. The child positions the diaper when lying on the side and then rolls backward on top of it so that the buttocks rest on the rear portion of the diaper. The child then sits up to grasp the front portion. Fastening the diaper tabs is best achieved by returning to lying. Since considerable practice may be required to fasten the tabs, the child should be encouraged to participate in this step as early as possible during training.

Donning Jackets and Front-Opening Shirts or Blouses   The child sits on the floor, or on a chair in front of a table. The garment is positioned wrong side up (its outer surface in contact with the floor or table) with the collar nearest the child. The child inserts his or her arms into the sleeves until the hands are visible at the other end. The arms are then raised overhead while the head ducks forward under the collar. The jacket or shirt should then fall into place on the child's back.

Adaptive Clothing

Careful selection or adaptation of clothing may make the difference between dependence and independence for the child. The following suggestions for modifying clothing have been offered by Nakos and Taylor (1977):

1. Long zippers sewn into the side seams of pants make it easier to slide the pants over braces or a catheter bag. When long-leg braces are worn under clothing, the pants should be one or two sizes larger than normal.
2. When buttons or zippers are difficult for the older child, Velcro fastenings can be substituted.
3. It is easier to place the feet into shoes that lace down to the toe. Sneakers with Velcro closures are useful for the young child who wears plastic lower-leg and foot orthoses and cannot tie shoelaces.

Bracing

Donning and Doffing Braces   Young children should be encouraged to assist in removing lower-extremity braces at the same time they begin to pull off shoes and socks. Most toddler-age children are able to participate by pulling tabs to undo Velcro fastenings and by lifting their legs out of the braces. The technique used to remove braces is determined by the type of braces and the child's abilities. Short- and long-leg braces are most easily removed in long sitting, whereas supine lying may be required when braces include a pelvic band.

To doff long-leg braces with a pelvic band, all straps are unfastened with the child in a sitting position. The child then removes the feet from the shoes and the legs from the lower portion of the braces. At this point, there are several options to complete the task. The child may roll to the side and then onto the abdomen, thus allowing the braces to slip off. Or the child may assume supine lying and lift the buttocks (bridging) while the braces are pulled from underneath.

The child should always be checked carefully for reddened areas after braces are removed. If reddening is present and persists for more than 15 minutes, it should be reported to the appropriate personnel for brace modification. Redness that does not disappear indicates that there is excessive pressure on the skin. Such areas may be at risk for skin breakdown and pressure sores. Generally, the preschool child does not have the judgment to examine the skin adequately. However, the caregiver should encourage the child of this age to assist in examining the skin.

The following is a step-by-step description for donning long-leg braces with a pelvic band, in a reclined or sitting position:

1. The adult should examine the child's skin before putting the braces on. If reddened areas are present, the braces should not be used prior to consulting with a physician or therapist.
2. The adult must be sure all fastenings are open and locks are disengaged. Shoes should be unlaced to the toe.
3. The adult should begin the donning process from the shoes and progress upward. The child's knees must be bent to get the feet into the shoes. When braces are of molded plastic, the adult should fit the child's foot into the brace before inserting it into the shoe.
4. The adult should check to ensure that the child's heels are down into the bottom of the shoes, and take care that toes are not curled inside the shoe. Some shoes have doubled tongues to hold the feet properly in the shoe. This inner support is tied first and should never be overlooked.
5. When buckling knee pads, the adult should keep the child's knees slightly flexed so that there will be room enough for the child to sit comfortably with knees bent.

6. The pelvic band should be buckled while the child is seated to allow for comfort in this position.

When it is difficult to distinguish left from right braces or shoes, they should be marked prior to home use. Commonly, braces are worn under outer clothing but over underwear and socks. It is not unusual, however, for some young children to wear braces over their pants.

The following guidelines are used to ensure the proper fit of braces:

1. The metal brace joints should be in line with the anatomical joints of the hips, knees, and ankles when the child stands in the braces.
2. The position of the metal uprights should be checked in standing. One finger should fit comfortably between the child's leg and the uprights.
3. When the child is seated, the pelvic band should not press against the groin area. There should also be room behind the knees to allow for skin folds. Neither the thigh cuff nor the calf cuff should press against the back of the knee.
4. Locks at hips and knees should slip down easily when the joint is extended (straightened). However, the locks on new braces may be initially stiff.
5. When new braces are acquired, the child should be frequently checked for reddened areas.
6. When a child has been wearing a pair of braces for an extended period, reddened areas may indicate the need for a larger size.

BATHING

In general, the infant with spina bifida can be bathed in the same way as any infant. Bath time provides an excellent opportunity for encouraging body awareness and play skills. The firm, deep pressure provided by washing and drying assists the child with full or partial sensation to become more aware of body parts. If sensation is absent, the caregiver can identify the body parts while encouraging the child to attend to them during bathing.

A nonslippery surface under the child, such as a baby bathmat or rubber kitchen sink mat, is helpful in providing a feeling of security for both the infant and the caregiver. When there is a high-level lesion, supporting the young infant during bathing is difficult. Sling bath seats with suction cups are commercially available to assist these children. The semireclined infant is then supported in a plastic net. As early as possible, the infant is encouraged to use one or both hands to squeeze a washcloth and to handle soap. Toys can be added to enhance the opportunity for play and learning.

As a child nears preschool age, active participation in the bathing process increases. This participation may not occur spontaneously in the child with spina bifida when sitting balance is poor. Proper positioning in the bathtub is therefore essential to free the hands for bathing. When a nonslip surface is insufficient for safety or when external trunk support is required, use of a tub seat should be considered. In selecting a suitable tub seat, care is necessary to ensure the proper height, width and depth of the seat. The following items are recommended for use as inexpensive bathtub seats:

1. A child-size lawn chair with aluminum frame and plastic webbing can be positioned in the tub on a nonslip rubber mat.
2. A small, inflatable ring inner tube can be used with the child seated in the middle of the ring or tube.
3. A meshed, plastic laundry basket can provide back and lateral support when the child is positioned within it.
4. A plastic laundry basket can be modified by cutting out one side. The child sits in the basket with legs extended. The cut edges of the basket are covered with plastic tape for safety. A rubber mat or towel is placed underneath the basket to prevent slippage.

Washing the hands and face is usually the first task in personal hygiene that the child learns. This skill can be easily practiced following mealtimes and during bathing. Additional experience is provided through play activities with a basin of water. As the child develops control, skill emerges in washing other body parts. With the exception of washing the hair, many children are independent in bathing at 4–5 years of age.

In the older child with spina bifida, self-bathing is dependent on the child's ability to get into and out of the bathtub safely and on the ability to reach freely during washing and drying. The child who is able to stand without braces can usually transfer in and out of the tub with the assistance of grab bars for support. If the legs cannot be lifted to step over the side of the tub, the child can sit on the edge of the tub, hold onto a grab bar with one hand, and assist the legs into the tub one at a time with the other hand. The grab bar is also used in lowering oneself to the bottom of the tub. A rubber bath mat is necessary for safety.

The child with a more severe disability may achieve independence by using a commercially available tub bench. The bench allows the child to transfer into a tub directly from a wheelchair and avoids having to lower the whole body down into the tub. Some tub benches have a back support to assist sitting balance. When using a tub bench, a shower hose is usually needed to bathe adequately. Self-bathing in a shower stall may be easier for some children, since it eliminates the need for transferring into and out of the tub. Use of a lawn chair or commercially available shower chair allows the hands to be free for bathing. When these suggestions are not sufficient to meet the child's physical needs, consultation with a therapist familiar with adaptive equipment is helpful in selecting the most appropriate techniques and adaptations for bathing.

Lack of sensation creates specific safety concerns regarding the temperature of the water. To prevent burns, it is essential that the child recognize the hot and cold water taps and be able to test the water temperature. The child must learn to test the temperature routinely with the hands before placing the legs into the water.

Bathing the legs is a typical problem encountered when movement of the lower extremities is minimal and sitting balance is difficult to maintain in a leaning forward position. A long-handled bath sponge allows the child to wash the legs and the back from the sitting position. The older child can use a shower hose for washing and rinsing the hard-to-reach areas including the hair. Nozzle heads are available with temperature controls. A glove or mitt washcloth is helpful for children with a weak grasp. Liquid soap can be used if handling a bar of soap is difficult.

BOWEL AND BLADDER MANAGEMENT

The nondisabled child approaching preschool age has usually achieved bowel and bladder control. However, since bowel and bladder functions are frequently affected in individuals with myelomeningocele, special management techniques may be required, from early infancy throughout adult life.

The Urinary System and Some Typical Problems

Proper functioning of the urinary system is a vital health issue for children with spina bifida. The nondisabled child empties the bladder completely numerous times a day by voluntarily contracting the bladder muscles when there is a feeling of fullness. The brain, spinal cord, and urinary system function in synchrony to provide voluntary control of bladder functioning. In spina bifida, this synchrony is frequently interrupted by a spinal cord lesion at or above the sacral area. Proper functioning of S-2, S-3, and S-4 spinal nerves is necessary for sensory awareness of bladder fullness, muscle tone of the bladder, and voluntary contraction of the bladder muscles. If this nerve supply is deficient, there is an inability to void in a controlled and voluntary manner, which results in a neurogenic bladder.

Some children have a flaccid bladder, in which the muscles of the bladder wall are hypotonic or limp. The relaxed muscles are unable to contract adequately to empty the bladder. Consequently, the bladder tends to remain full, with overflow of urine occurring in an uncontrolled, dribbling fashion. Other children have a spastic bladder that is irritable and tight. The bladder does not serve as a storage area, since the hypertonic muscles involuntarily contract causing leakage. Retention of residual urine in the bladder, causing susceptibility to infection, can occur in either the flaccid or spastic condition.

The urinary system is composed of two kidneys, which filter water-soluble waste from the blood and produce urine. Attached to each kidney is a tube, the ureter, that carries the urine to a balloon-like sack, the bladder, for storage. From the bladder, a single tube, the urethra, transports the urine for elimination—via the end of the penis in the male; above the entrance to the vagina in the female. Sphincter muscles control the flow from the bladder to the urethra. Under normal conditions, when the bladder is distended due to the accumulation of urine, the muscles of the bladder contract and the sphincter muscles relax, allowing the urine to escape through the urethra.

In spina bifida, the normal coordination of the bladder and sphincter muscles may be defective. The sphincter fails to open adequately as the weak bladder muscles contract. As a result, residual urine remains in the bladder after voiding, and urinary tract infections may occur. An additional problem can develop when urine in the full bladder backs up into the ureters, causing urinary reflux. In this condition, the ureters can become harmfully enlarged, and the kidneys can be damaged from the urinary pressure and infection. Renal (kidney) deterioration can be a life-threatening consequence in severe cases.

Urological Assessment

Proper bladder management begins with regular urological assessment, starting in infancy. At the outset, various tests are commonly performed to determine the type and degree of urological deficit and to manage its course over time. A *cystometrogram* is a study of the functional ability of the bladder. As a mild saline solution is introduced into the bladder, graphic recordings are obtained of the muscle contractions of the bladder wall in response to stretch. A *cystogram* is a test to detect reflux of urine into the ureters. After being filled with a radio-opaque fluid, the bladder is x-rayed in order to determine its size and shape. In a *cystoscopic examination,* the interior of the bladder is viewed through a cystoscope (a small tube with a lighted end that is inserted into the bladder).

An *intravenous pyelogram* (IVP) is an x-ray procedure that provides information on the anatomy of the ureters and the function of the kidneys. Analysis of the quantity of urea nitrogen in the blood can also provide an indication of kidney function. A *urinalysis* is a laboratory examination of the urine that includes a culture to determine the presence of bacteria.

In general, recommendations are made for high fluid intake to assist the urinary flow, since residual urine in the bladder fosters growth of bacteria and infection. Cranberry juice is often suggested, as it alters the pH of urine and helps to prevent bladder stone formation. Special diet recommendations may also be given by the physician.

Urinary tract infection (cystitis) is rather common in children with spina bifida. Therefore, a urine culture should be conducted on a quarterly basis during the first 2 years of life and bi-annually thereafter (Kass, 1982). When an infection occurs, antibiotic therapy is used in combination with techniques for bladder management. Since a urinary tract infection can occur at any time, it is important for all adults involved with the child to be familiar with its symptoms. When signs of infection are detected during school hours, the school nurse and the child's parents should be alerted. One should remember that a fever in a child with myelomeningocele more frequently indicates a urinary tract infection than a nose or throat infection. Warning signs of a urinary tract infection may include a low-grade temperature, a cloudy or dark colored appearance to the urine, odorous urine, general fatigue, and nausea.

It is recommended that the young child receive a complete urological evaluation on a regular basis. Once the type and degree of deficit is determined, a multidisciplinary team assists the family in carrying out the appropriate techniques for the child's bladder management. The team nurse is frequently responsible for teaching appropriate techniques and serves as the liaison between the parents and the team. The major emphases in urological management are preservation of renal function and control of incontinence. Over the past 15 years, a variety of management techniques, both conservative and surgical, have been developed that are geared toward reducing the amount of residual urine in the bladder and facilitating urinary outflow.

Bladder Management Techniques

The following is a brief description of current methods of bladder management as they pertain to the preschool- and school-age child.

The Crede Maneuver   In the Crede Maneuver, external manual pressure is applied in a downward direction on the lower abdomen (over the bladder) to assist bladder drainage. It is often taught to parents to encourage their infant's complete bladder emptying at each diaper change. Many children can be taught to "crede" the bladder independently; the younger child should be encouraged to perform the technique with adult supervision. Though continence is rarely achieved by use of this method alone, it reduces residual urine and the chances of infection.

Internal Collecting Devices   An indwelling catheter is a small tube that is inserted through the urethra into the bladder to achieve urinary drainage. It is also used to prevent backflow of urine into the kidneys. The tube is attached to a collecting bag strapped to the inside of the child's leg, which can be emptied as needed. This device can be worn by males or females. If the necessary cognitive, perceptual, and fine motor skills are present, the child can learn to empty the collecting bag independently. However, long-term use of an indwelling catheter is generally not recommended.

External Collecting Devices   In males with adequate penile size, a condom-type sheath can be worn that is attached by a flexible tube to a collecting bag. The most commonly used appliance is a Texas catheter. Since no suitable external device has been developed for females, they may need to use cellulose padding and rubber pants.

Intermittent Catheterization   A major advance in the management of the neurogenic bladder is the use of intermittent nonsterile self-catheterization. Children using this technique tend to stay dry and maintain stable renal function when a strictly timed catheterization schedule is followed (Carlson & Stone, 1982). Frequently, medication is required as an adjunct to this method (Kass, 1982). Anticholinergic drugs (e.g., Ditropan, Probanthine) may be employed to expand the storage capacity of the bladder; alpha adrenergic drugs (e.g., ephedrine, Ornade) may be prescribed to decrease urinary dribbling.

Intermittent catheterization involves the insertion of a rubber, metal, or soft plastic tube (catheter) through the urethra into the bladder. Complete emptying of the bladder is achieved by the urine flowing out of the catheter into a receptacle or toilet. The catheter must be clean, but sterile conditions are not necessary. Catheterization is usually performed every 2–4 hours, at regular intervals. It is most important to adhere to the schedule in order to prevent urinary complications.

The procedure can be introduced during infancy and can be performed independently by most children by 7 or 8 years of age. Many preschool children can learn the technique if they are motivated and have quality instruction and practice. It may be difficult, however, to teach self-catheterization to the preschool child who has cognitive or preceptual-motor deficits secondary to hydrocephalus (Hannigan, 1979).

Surgical Approaches The success of intermittent catheterization has markedly decreased the need for permanent urinary diversion through surgical procedures (Borzyskowski, 1984; Riggs, 1982). Indeed, surgical approaches to the management of the neurogenic bladder are seldom conducted with young children unless more conservative methods have failed to protect against damage to the kidneys. When a surgical approach is indicated, a section of intestine is used to divert the flow of urine to an opening (stoma) in the abdominal wall. A collecting bag is fitted around the stoma with adhesive. Continence is achieved by the urine draining into the bag, which is emptied at regular intervals.

Care of the stoma is important to prevent leakage and skin irritation. Symptoms of possible problems with the urinary diversion include elevation in temperature, pain at the stoma, blood in the urine, and a decreased output of urine. In general, there are no restrictions to the child's activity as a consequence of this procedure. The use of an artificial sphincter, surgically implanted to control urinary incontinence, is presently gaining attention. This approach is employed more frequently with adolescents and adults than with children.

Bowel Management Techniques

Bowel incontinence is frequently associated with spina bifida. Many children do not have the sensation and control needed to defecate volitionally. Therefore, toilet training in the sense that it is usually understood is not relevant. Instead, a bowel management program involves toileting at regularly scheduled times. By adhering to a set routine, a regime is established for bowel movement, generally on a daily basis. A consistent routine is important to avoid accidents. Diapering may be a necessary adjunct for the child who is unable to maintain a predictable management schedule. As the child grows older, diapers can be purchased in large sizes, and various undergarments are available with disposable liners.

A bowel management program includes monitoring the dietary intake, preventing constipation, and evacuation of the bowels on a regular basis (Frank & Fixsen, 1980). Although a few children are troubled with loose, uncontrolled passage of stool, most have problems of constipation. Retained stool can result over time in harmful dilation of the colon. A diet high in fiber content and roughage is often recommended, emphasizing cereals with bran, nuts, mixed vegetables, and certain fruits (Shepherd, Hickstein, & Shepherd, 1983). Prune juice is commonly used as a bowel stimulant. At times, stool softeners such as Senokot and Cologel are prescribed, and suppositories may be used to achieve proper timing of the bowel movement.

Summary

There are no easy solutions to bowel and bladder incontinence in children with spina bifida. This fact creates stress for parents and professionals; but most important, it is distressing to the child. With age, the child starts to assist with personal hygiene, learns to empty collecting bags, or begins to self-catheterize (Okamoto et al., 1984). However, many children will continue to need assistance with bowel and bladder management. Most preschoolers will be at least partially dependent on adults for diapering and catheterization.

During the preschool years, children begin to be aware of their differences in comparison to their peers. This is therefore the time to address their feelings regarding problems of incontinence. The children will need understanding and support to alleviate the anxiety and embarrassment that can result from bowel and bladder dysfunction.

FEEDING AND DIET

The development of feeding skills is important for the child's physical, emotional, and social development. The presence of feeding problems may interfere with intake of the food necessary for health, adequate nutrition, and general well-being. The feeding problems observed in some children with spina bifida are not unique to this population, but are common among children with developmental disabilities. They include difficulties in achieving proper positioning at mealtime, deficiencies in oral-motor control, and delays in the development of hand use for self-feeding. Obesity is a common issue and one that may require special management of the diet.

The following discussion includes an overview of the normal development of feeding skills—including positioning, oral-motor control, and self-feeding.

Familiarity with normal patterns may assist the parent and clinician in recognizing problems that may interfere with skill acquisition. Common problems are then described, with accompanying suggestions for intervention.

Positioning for Feeding

As a child develops, positions for feeding are modified in accordance with the child's development of postural control. The newborn infant requires support of the head and trunk and is usually fed while totally supported in the caregiver's arms. The infant is held with the head slightly forward and the trunk in a semireclined position. The forward posture of the head facilitates swallowing as well as decreasing the likelihood of aspiration and choking on fluid. This position also enables the child and caregiver to engage readily in social interaction.

As the child grows, holding him or her in the arms during feeding becomes cumbersome, although sufficient trunk control for the child to sit independently may not be present. At this time, the child may be fed in an infant seat, which offers a semireclined, supported position. The nondisabled child has sufficient head control by approximately 3–4 months to maintain the head slightly forward during feeding. As the child achieves independent sitting with good trunk control, readiness is demonstrated for feeding in a highchair or booster seat.

Because of physical limitations, the child with myelomeningocele may require some modifications in positioning. For example, at birth, the infant may need to be fed while lying on his or her abdomen, with the head supported on the caregiver's lap and turned to the side. This position is commonly used both pre- and postoperatively to prevent pressure or irritation to the site of the lesion. The position, however, makes feeding more difficult for some infants and decreases the opportunity for the child to engage in social activity during the process. Feeding time may then be a less pleasurable experience for both child and caregiver.

Depending on the level of lesion, the child with spina bifida may have poor development of head and trunk control, which influences the selection of a feeding position. Chapter 5 provides general suggestions for intervention when there is a need to modify the child's position or provide external support. Additional considerations pertaining to feeding are presented in this discussion.

The child's head posture should be closely observed. If the head is tilted back (hyperextended) during feeding, swallowing is difficult and choking results. The following suggestions may be helpful to achieve a slight forward placement of the head when the child is being fed in an infant seat:

1. A small pillow may be placed behind the infant's head.
2. The adult should be at eye level with the child during feeding. When the adult is positioned above the child, head hyperextension is encouraged as the child attempts to look up at the caregiver.

3. The bottle or spoon should be introduced from a direction below the mouth. As the child looks down toward the food, a proper head position is reinforced.

If the child lacks control to keep the head in midline, a small pillow or rolled towel can be placed on either side of the head to maintain a midline orientation. An older child with a strabismus may demonstrate head tilting in order to focus on the food during self-feeding. This type of head tilt allows the child to be functional and should not be confused with poor head control. At times, the child with poor trunk control sits with an excessively rounded back; during feeding, the head tilts backward as the child looks up to eat. In such cases, a slightly reclined seat may be used to achieve better alignment of the head and trunk and to avoid neck hyperextension.

In addition to concern for proper posture, one should be aware of the position of the child's arms. In general, the arms should be placed forward in front of the body. In preparation for self-feeding, the hands are placed on utensils and guided to the mouth with the caregiver's assistance. The child's other hand is used to stabilize the plate or bowl.

Oral-Motor Function

Oral-motor function refers to the ability to control the oral musculature in order to suck, swallow, remove food from a spoon, and chew. In each of these actions, movements of the tongue, lips, and jaw are combined in a coordinated manner for normal nutritional intake.

Normal Feeding Patterns   During the first few months of life, the rooting reflex assists the infant to obtain food. As soon as the nipple touches the lips or side of the cheek, the infant immediately turns toward the stimulus, opens the mouth, and begins to suckle. The efficiency of the suckling pattern enables most infants to ingest 6–8 ounces of liquid from a bottle in approximately 20–30 minutes (Morris, 1981).

Gradually, the initial suckling pattern, which is reflexive in nature, develops into a more voluntarily controlled pattern. This change usually occurs with the introduction of semisolid foods from a spoon. Pureed foods are commonly given at 3–6 months, depending on the advice of the pediatrician. Since spoon feeding is a new experience for the infant, there may be some coughing or gagging initially. The child may need to pause and may indicate this by turning the head. This stage frequently coincides with feeding in a more upright position in an infant seat.

Generally between 6 and 9 months, the infant is able to coordinate the lips, tongue, and jaw in order to manage more solid foods. The child may suck on a cookie at 6 months but gradually progress to a munching pattern. Munching entails an up-and-down movement of the jaw and tongue to chew such foods as graham crackers or cooked carrots. During this time, the infant's lip control improves for removal of food from a spoon and the beginning of assisted cup drinking. In the early cup-drinking period, the child uses one to three sucks for every swallow while coordinating this sequence with breathing. Initially, the tongue moves with the jaw in an up-and-down fashion while drinking. The child may firmly press the cup against the corners of the lips to reduce the loss of liquid or bite the cup to obtain stability of the jaw.

During the 12–18 month period, the movement of the lips, tongue, and jaw become more selective, with each moving more independently (the process of dissociation). The child bites off and chews pieces of food such as meat, fresh fruits, cooked vegetables, and crackers. Rotary movements of the jaw are observed in a more mature chewing pattern. Lateral movements of the tongue allow for proper positioning of food between the teeth for chewing. In cup drinking, the child drinks for longer periods without stopping; and because of improved jaw stabilization, there is little loss of liquid. During this time, the child may begin to use gestures or single words to indicate food preferences, hunger, or satiation.

Oral-Motor Dysfunction and Hypersensitivity   Feeding patterns can be considered immature or primitive when the child does not achieve the oral-motor function expected for a specific age level. *Primitive* feeding patterns may be related to general developmental delay, oral hypersensitivity, or lack of experience with managing more solid food. In contrast, *abnormal* patterns are associated with damage to the central nervous system and are never seen in the physically intact infant. They include a tonic tongue thrust, tonic bite reflex, pathological jaw thrusting, and spastic lip or tongue retraction.

Most commonly, the feeding difficulties of some children with spina bifida are related to hypersensitivity around the oral area and delayed or poor oral-motor control. The occurrence of abnormal oral-motor patterns secondary to brain damage is less common except in severely impaired children with hydrocephalus. Consequently, this discussion does not address specific intervention for pathological oral dysfunction. Therapy for this condition is described extensively in the professional literature (Connor et al., 1978; Finnie, 1975; Morris, 1977).

Oral hypersensitivity is the inability to tolerate touch or other sensory stimulation in or near the mouth. When confronted with a stimulus, the orally hypersensitive child may exhibit general withdrawal reactions, such as excessive startling, irritability, or changes in muscle tone. These behaviors frequently occur when the mouth is stimulated by a bottle, cup, spoon, or item of food; it may also be noted when the child's face is touched with a hand or washcloth. The following behaviors may indicate more specifically the presence of hypersensitivity of the oral area:

1. Turning the face away from the breast or bottle despite the infant being hungry

2. Facial grimacing when touched on the face
3. Spitting out of food
4. Tight closing of the lips on presentation of semisolid or solid foods
5. Poor adjusting to varied food textures and temperatures
6. Excessive gagging

The presence of hypersensitivity can interfere with the normal acquisition of feeding skills and the social interactions that occur during mealtimes. Rather than being a positive experience, mealtimes are difficult and frustrating for the child and parent. There may be a reluctance to introduce foods of varied textures due to fear of gagging. Yet when solid foods are not introduced, the development of refined movements of the tongue, lips, and jaw may be delayed, and feeding patterns may remain immature.

The following activities may be helpful in decreasing oral hypersensitivity. Consultation with a specially trained therapist working with the child is important in determining the appropriate type of intervention. These activities can be conducted just prior to feeding or in the course of daily routines.

1. The adult should gradually increase the amount of tactile stimulation tolerated by the child. This is begun with the trunk, since touch of this area is usually acceptable to the child. The adult holds the child firmly and provides total body contact while rocking. Firm, deep pressure should be used rather than a light touch, which the child may find irritating. "Roughhousing" can increase the child's tolerance when presented at an appropriate level.
2. Play with various textures such as water, sand, or paint should be encouraged.
3. The adult should gradually increase tolerance for touch on the face by having the infant experience the feel of soft rubber toys in or near the mouth, or by encouraging the infant to bring the hands to the face for exploration. The adult can apply firm pressure with the hand or a soft cloth around the cheeks and mouth, by rubbing or patting slowly in one direction using firm pressure.
4. When the child can accept general stimulation, one can concentrate on the intra-oral area. The adult can firmly rub the gums from the side to the midline with the index finger. Placing pleasant-tasting food on the finger while working in the child's mouth will provide a pleasurable taste sensation.

To reduce sensitivity to foods, one should gradually move from pureed foods to table food and increase experience with varied temperatures and tastes. The following progression is suggested:

Pureed foods

Thicker foods and liquids, such as mashed potatoes, oatmeal, yogurt, eggnog, or vegetable juice

Granular semisolids, such as scrambled eggs, cottage cheese, mashed bananas, or rice pudding

Transitional foods that are firm and chewy, such as cheese, cooked but firm carrots, bread, or pieces of meat or chicken

Individual diets may preclude the use of certain suggested foods. For example, cheese intake may be limited due to its calcium content. The use of sweet foods and drinks may also be restricted, since they frequently increase drooling and contribute to unwanted weight gain. It is important to enable the child to progress gradually but systematically to a diet of diversely textured solid foods in order to decrease hypersensitivity and to promote mature movement patterns of the oral area.

Self-Feeding

Normal Patterns of Self-Feeding   Self-feeding is a complex task requiring the integration of perceptual systems with controlled movement of the oral area and upper limb. Precursor skills to self-feeding are noted in early hand-to-mouth behaviors, such as sucking the hand for self-consolation or mouthing objects and toys. Finger feeding emerges around 7 months. In the earliest stage of finger feeding, the infant may hold the biscuit in a forced grip. Over subsequent months, the child's grasp pattern refines to the point where small pieces of food can be lifted using only the thumb and index finger. However, excessive force may be used, and release in the mouth is still crude. Usually by 1 year of age, the child demonstrates greater control in holding and releasing finger foods.

Skill in managing a bottle independently is also acquired developmentally. An infant first holds a bottle and brings it to the mouth at 6 months, using the fingers to press the bottle against the palms and requiring a degree of adult assistance for lifting the bottle. In the months that follow, grasp patterns on the bottle mature. By 10 months, the child is actively reaching for, grasping, and directing the bottle to the mouth independently. When cup drinking is introduced, spilling is a common occurrence. Spilling is related to difficulty in maintaining a hold on the cup, grading movement of the cup to the mouth, and controlling the speed of the liquid's flow. Cup drinking is usually not mastered until 2 years of age.

A developmental progression is also noted in the use of eating utensils. As early as 8–9 months, the child begins to guide the caregiver's hand in feeding with a spoon. Just as grasp patterns mature for finger feeding and bottle drinking, changes in the grasp of utensils are observed over time. At 15 months, the child initiates holding the spoon in a fisted hand with the palm facing down (pronation of the forearm). As the hand is brought to the mouth, spilling occurs because the hand turns down. Gradually, the child learns to hold the spoon between the thumb and fingers as well as to place the spoon properly into the mouth (through controlled supination of the forearm). Although the child may be successful at self-feeding semisolid and solid foods with a spoon by 3–4 years, it is not until 6 years of age that the child becomes proficient in managing liquids, such as soups, with a spoon.

The grasp of a fork develops in an identical pattern. At approximately 4½ years of age, the child has had sufficient experience with both spoon and fork to be able to choose correctly one over the other, depending on the type of food. The knife is the last utensil to be introduced. The child manages the knife using a fisted grasp with the index finger extended toward the blade end. This grasp remains the same for both spreading and cutting, although the orientation of the knife differs. For spreading, which begins at approximately 6 years of age, the knife is held with the blade turned to the side. For cutting, which begins at approximately 7 years, the knife is held with the blade side down. When cutting or spreading, the opposite hand is usually used to stabilize the food, either with or without a fork.

Problems in Self-Feeding   The child with spina bifida may encounter difficulty with self-feeding if a deficit exists in oral-motor control, coordination of the upper extremity, visual perception, and/or motor planning. The importance of oral-motor control has already been addressed in this chapter, and its role in self-feeding is obvious. If skilled manipulation of the arms is lacking, the child may have difficulty achieving mature grasp patterns on utensils, putting food on utensils, bringing food to the mouth without spilling, and stabilizing food on the plate for effective cutting and spreading. If visual-motor skills or motor planning are deficient, the child may have difficulty planning the movement sequence required to put food on a fork or spoon or to use a knife effectively.

Chapter 6 provides intervention strategies to improve perceptual-motor development. When evaluating self-feeding skills, it is necessary to determine which specific areas are impeding function in order to determine what types of intervention will be most successful. The following activities may also be helpful in promoting self-feeding skills:

1. Encouraging hand-to-mouth behavior in early infancy.
2. Encouraging placement of hands on the bottle or breast during feeding.
3. Using a Tommie Tippie or weighted cup to reduce the incidence of spills.
4. Introduction of spoon feeding using the following special technique to increase control of the hand-to-mouth pattern. The adult sits at the side of the child and holds the spoon with the index and middle fingers of the same hand extended along its handle. The child grasps the adult's two fingers, which serve as a built-up handle on the spoon. During feeding, the adult

can provide very specific guidance to the child's upper extremity based on the child's needs. This procedure allows fine gradations of the child's elbow, forearm, and wrist motions. The child experiences more controlled assistance using this technique than in the more traditional hand-over-hand method.

5. Using a wide or built-up handle on a utensil when the child's grasp is weak.
6. Presenting foods in a graded manner when frequent spilling with a spoon is a problem. The adult should begin with sticky foods, progress to looser semisolids, and last, introduce liquids.
7. Providing scoop dishes with steep sides for the child who initially has difficulty scooping food onto a spoon.
8. Progressing from soft to hard solids if the child has weak muscle strength for cutting with a knife.
9. Using suction cups or nonslip place mats under plates if the child cannot stabilize the plate while eating.

Oral Hygiene

Of special concern is the need to establish early patterns of good oral hygiene. This can be achieved in infancy by cleansing the gums and early teeth with gauze tightly wrapped around the adult's index finger (Haynes, 1983). The gauze is dipped in a saline solution before being used to massage the oral area. This solution is made by dissolving ½ teaspoon of salt in 8 ounces of water. (Caution is required to ensure that the gauze does not slip down the child's throat.)

The young child with oral-motor defensiveness may be resistant to having his or her teeth brushed by an adult. Introducing brushing of the teeth into the daily routine as early as teeth are present is generally helpful. If the young child is orally hypersensitive and is fearful of a toothbrush, the gauze massaging technique can be used as a substitute. In general, supervised independent brushing of the teeth is emphasized between 3 and 4 years of age. Practice for this activity is provided by having the child imitate brushing with a small toothbrush. Hand-over-hand assistance by an adult is usually necessary in the beginning. If grasp of the toothbrush is difficult, the handle may be built up with rubber or foam tubing, to enable the child to grasp it more effectively. An electric toothbrush may assist in the proper dental care of some older children.

Diet

The child with spina bifida may exhibit secondary medical complications that can be minimized through proper nutrition and diet. These concerns include osteoporosis, urological problems, and obesity. In the case of osteoporosis, there is increased porosity of the bones that causes them to soften and be more vulnerable to fracture. Osteoporosis is characterized by bone resorption (the loss of calcium from the bones) and can occur as a result of low activity and an absence of weight bearing. Pressure on the bones through the support of body weight and use of the muscles appears to stimulate bone calcium deposit. In the case of bed confinement or marked restriction in activity, calcium deposit may become overbalanced by calcium resorption. In the presence of osteoporosis, a diet high in calcium and Vitamin D may be recommended to aid in improved calcification of the bones.

However, the loss of bone calcium is also associated with an increase in the calcium concentration in the urine. This increased concentration may result in the development of kidney and bladder stones, for which a low-calcium diet is recommended (Williams, 1981). Thus, it is important that a physician and clinical dietician be consulted to determine the type of diet that is most appropriate for a particular child.

Obesity is a common problem in infants and young children with spina bifida, due in part to their physical inactivity. Weight-for-age charts may underestimate the degree of obesity, since these children are commonly short in stature compared to nondisabled peers. Even the standard weight-for-height criteria may be misleading. In children with myelomeningocele, body fat constitutes a comparatively larger proportion of body mass because of the decrease in muscle tissue and increase in fat of the lower extremities (Rickard et al., 1977). Excessive weight gain during childhood often becomes a major weight control problem by adolescence.

Nutritional screening and management are important to prevent the child from becoming overweight. Sound eating habits should be established early, and weight should be carefully monitored. Restricted intake is advisable of high-calorie, low-nutrient foods such as cake, candy, carbonated beverages, and synthetic drinks. Cranberry juice diluted with water is a good alternative to synthetic drinks for children requiring high fluid intake to prevent kidney infections and constipation.

A frequent component of a bowel management program is inclusion in the diet of foods with high fiber content to minimize constipation. These foods include whole grain breads, bran, green leafy vegetables, and fruits whose peel can be eaten, such as apples.

Mealtime as a Social Experience

Mealtimes provide a social and communicative experience for the child and parent, starting in infancy. When the infant cries in hunger, the adult responds with food. The baby is generally held close to the caregiver's body and hears the voice and sees the face of the adult. The child becomes more relaxed and satisfied as the meal progresses. This situation is positive and rewarding for both participants.

However, when a young infant has a feeding problem, a different set of communicative interactions may occur. The child with spina bifida may need to be held in some other position during feeding on account of surgery or poor head and trunk control, thus providing less satisfying physical contact with the adult. Such problems as hypersensitivity in the oral area or weak suckling may contribute to irritability and frustration. The parent may feel inadequate and may unintentionally relate this tension to the child. As a result of such factors, feeding may become an unpleasant time for all.

Early identification of feeding difficulties and the subsequent management of those difficulties enhance feelings of competence for both child and caregiver. Through the proper positioning and intervention strategies previously described, mealtimes can become a mutually gratifying experience.

TRANSFERS

Assisting with Transfers

One of the most important considerations in transferring a child is the use of good body mechanics. The adult's proper use of his or her body minimizes the possibility of muscle strain while lifting and allows a smooth, safe transfer. The following recommendations should be kept in mind by the individual assisting the transfer:

1. The adult should properly position the child and wheelchair prior to beginning the actual transfer. The wheelchair should always be locked during a transfer.
2. The child's weight and size should be assessed, allowing for the weight of the braces. If the child is too heavy for one individual to manage, the transfer should be performed by two people.
3. The adult's feet should be spaced comfortably apart in a step position. There is then a wide base of support with the ability to shift weight in any direction.
4. The adult should keep the child as close to the body as possible. The child's body weight is then supported by the adult's skeletal frame and not by excessive muscular effort.
5. The adult should keep the back straight and always bend at the knees when lifting. The adult must not lean over at the hips with stiff legs, and lift the child by arching the low back. The legs should perform the work in the lift.
6. The adult should avoid twisting the trunk during the transfer, since this causes loss of control and muscular strain.

Maximum participation of the child should always be encouraged, thus working toward the ultimate goal of independence in transferring. The degree of participation is influenced by the child's age, cognitive level, muscle strength, and motivation. These factors are also pertinent in selecting the appropriate type of transfer to be employed.

A dependent transfer technique is used when the child requires total assistance in moving from one surface to another because of his or her age or motor handicap. The child is actually lifted and carried. With the young child, this type of assistance is frequently required in transferring from a low to a high surface, such as from the floor to a chair. A dependent transfer of the young child can generally be performed by one person, although special circumstances may require the assistance of two individuals.

If the child is to be carried, two approaches can be used to lift the child. The adult can be positioned behind the child or at the side. Either approach should incorporate the recommendations previously listed for proper use of the body. It is also important to provide external support for the child's lower extremities to prevent injury. A child wearing braces has the support needed to maintain the legs in adequate alignment. A child without braces needs the support of the adult's arm or arms to maintain the legs in a neutral, well-aligned posture.

In lifting the child from behind, the adult stoops by bending at the knees. The child is held under the buttocks and upper thighs, close to the adult. The adult then rises, using his or her leg muscles. If the child is to be lifted from the floor, the adult may choose a kneeling position behind the child. After securing the child with the arms, the adult moves into a half-kneeling position while keeping the back straight, then proceeds to standing. When lifting from the side, the adult places one arm under the child's thighs and the other arm around the upper back of the child in a corralling fashion.

A two-person transfer may be required when the child is wearing postsurgical long-leg casts. One lifter stands behind the child and holds him or her around the chest below the arms. The second lifter stands facing the child and raises the child's lower body by supporting under the thighs. Since most of the weight in a two-person lift is borne by the adult behind the child, it is recommended that the stronger individual assume this placement.

The following transfers can be performed independently or with assistance. In learning to transfer by themselves, children will require varying degrees of help. It is important that the transfer routine be consistent each time it is practiced. When teaching the child to transfer or when assisting in transfers, the adult should carefully consider the amount of assistance required for the transfer to be safe.

Transfer Techniques

Sliding Board Transfer The sliding board transfer is performed in a sitting position using a smooth wooden board to move from one surface to another. It is most appropriate for the nonambulatory child who is able to maintain sitting balance by using the arms, without external support. The child must have enough arm strength to push up on straight arms and slide the body across the surface of the board. The technique can be used for transferring into and out of a wheelchair, into a car, or onto a tub bench, a bed, or another chair. With the young child, the transferring surfaces need to be fairly equal in height.

Unequal heights require greater adult assistance, since the child must slide on an inclined board.

1. Prior to transfer, the wheelchair's armrest and legrest are removed from the side on which the transfer is to be performed. The wheelchair is positioned alongside the transfer surface and as close as possible to it. Since the sliding board serves as a bridge between the two surfaces, the distance can be no greater than approximately two-thirds the length of the board. The wheelchair is then locked.
2. One end of the sliding board is placed under the child's buttocks, the other end on the surface onto which the child is transferring. The child then slides, using both arms to push down on the board. Assistance by the adult can be provided from behind the chair.

A sliding board can also be utilized to help an adult effect the dependent transfer of a child. The board holds most of the child's body weight, freeing the adult to slide the child from one surface to the other.

Stand-Pivot Transfer The stand-pivot transfer requires that the child be able to support some weight on the legs, either with or without braces. When the child has good arm strength, this transfer can be performed independently. It can be employed by the nonambulatory child for transfers from a wheelchair to a toilet, bed, tub bench, or other seat. The presence of braces generally eases the transfer by externally supporting the legs.

1. The wheelchair is positioned as close as possible to the transfer surface, usually at a right angle to it.
2. The legrests are removed from the wheelchair, and the feet are positioned flat on the floor.
3. The child pushes on the armrests of the wheelchair to a standing position and switches one hand from the wheelchair to the other surface. (If transferring toward the right, the child would lead with the right hand.)
4. The child pivots, turning the body so as to be able to sit directly on the other surface. Assistance may be required when the child pushes up toward standing and pivots on the feet before sitting down again.

Forward and Backward Transfers Forward and backward transfers are useful in the home for moving onto or off of a bed. For the more skilled child, they can also be used for transfers into or out of a car. Similar to a sliding board transfer, these transfers require adequate arm strength and sitting balance. The technique necessitates that one of the two surfaces involved in the transfer must be large enough to support the child in long sitting (legs straight out in front of the child). The following is the procedure for forward transfer from the wheelchair to the bed (procedure is reversed to transfer backward into the wheelchair):

1. The wheelchair is positioned facing the bed. Legrests are removed or swung to the sides. Both legs are lifted onto the bed. The wheelchair is then finally positioned and locked.

2. The child pushes down with the arms several times in succession, moving forward each time. Care is taken to raise the buttocks so as to prevent skin injury, rather than to drag the buttocks forward across the surface. Thus, the child progresses onto the bed in a long-sitting position.

Wheelchair/Floor Transfer   Stable stools, graduated in height, are used as steps to bridge the distance between the wheelchair and the floor. The following is the procedure for transferring from the wheelchair to the floor:

1. The wheelchair is positioned behind the highest stool in the set of "steps."

2. The child proceeds in a manner similar to the forward transfer, but considerable arm strength is required to lower the buttocks forward gently on the steps. With many children, a program of upper-extremity strengthening is needed to prepare for this technique. The muscles controlling shoulder girdle depression (e.g., the latissimus dorsi) are particularly important for executing this transfer.

The procedure is reversed for transfer from floor to wheelchair. The child is positioned on the floor at the base of the first step with his or her back toward the chair. The child places the hands behind on the stool and pushes down to lift the buttocks backward onto the stool. To assist this progression, the pushing down is performed with a simultaneous tucking of the chin toward the chest. For the older child with good balance and arm strength, this transfer can be accomplished with only one stool as an intermediate step.

◇ CHAPTER 9 ◇

Special Considerations for the Classroom

EARLY CHILDHOOD EXPERIENCES PROVIDE A FOUNDATION FOR LATER LEARNing and influence the child's life outcome. The educational environment for the child with spina bifida need not be markedly different from any preschool classroom. Indeed, the goal is for the child to participate in as normal a social and educational setting as possible. Whether in a regular or special class, the curriculum of a state-of-the-art preschool program is based on the premise that the young child is an active learner and a spontaneous explorer.

This chapter discusses the nature of the preschool curriculum, strategies for designing opportunities to promote learning, methods to expand self-care skills in the classroom, and gross motor activities appropriate for a group setting. The discussion builds on the information presented in previous chapters in order to focus on the special requirements of the preschool class.

THE PRESCHOOL CURRICULUM

The preschool curriculum (for children 3–4 years of age) spans intervention in four major areas: cognition, communication, physical development, and psychosocial skills. Activities are provided for the development of self-care and adaptive skills, receptive and expressive language, sensory and perceptual processing, strength and coordination in gross and fine motor tasks, academic readiness skills, and interactional play. Strategies for implementing the preschool program include individual, small-group, and class instruction; active exploration and use of materials; free play; individual and small-group therapy sessions; and field trips.

During the preschool years, the child with spina bifida usually requires the services of an interdisciplinary team working in close collaboration with the parents. It is critical that goals and objectives for intervention be cooperatively developed to achieve an integrated program for the child. Mutually agreed upon goals and strategies ensure program implementation at home and in school, and facilitate the generalization of learning. Ongoing communication with the parents is strengthened by individual conferences, routine phone contacts, parent observation in the classroom, and home visits.

Coping: A Key Ingredient for Learning

In addition to activities that foster the acquisition of specific developmental skills, the curriculum should provide activities that promote the child's ability to cope effectively. Coping is the active process of using one's resources to meet personal needs and to adapt to the demands of the environment in ways that maintain or enhance feelings of well-being. Coping by the young child to meet personal needs involves the fulfillment of basic requirements for nutrition, security, a balance of activity and rest, as well as responding to preferences and the innate drive to achieve mastery. Coping to meet the demands of the environment requires the child to manage the physical surroundings, interact with objects, and adapt to social conditions.

Coping behaviors are learned through transactions with the world. The child's constitutional characteristics and interactions with the environment contribute to a unique coping style that reflects the way the child habitually uses certain strategies rather than others to manage the world. Based upon a longitudinal study of the development of coping competence from infancy to adolescence, Murphy and Moriarty (1976) have identified major elements that influence the acquisition of coping behaviors: the child's development, temperament, prior experience, areas of vulnerability, and the demands of the environment.

Since coping is an adaptive, learned process, coping behaviors are acquired and changed through experience (Moos, 1976; Zeitlin, 1981a). A child draws upon both internal and external resources to develop a variety of management strategies that can be applied to specific situations as coping efforts. The child's internal resources include physical health and neurological status, developmental competence, coping behavior patterns, and emerging beliefs about oneself and the world. These beliefs shape the child's perception of events. External resources are factors of the physical and social environment that support the child's coping efforts and provide opportunities for exploration and learning.

Coping is a process; it does not imply success, but effort. The effectiveness of one's coping behavior is determined by the "goodness of fit" or match between the child's actions and the situational demands (Lazarus & Folkman, 1984). Goodness of fit results when expectations and environmental demands are in accord with the child's resources. It does not imply an absence of stress and conflict, but rather the availability of resources to manage them. Poorness of fit can occur if environmental demands and expectations are excessive, even for a child with normally adequate resources.

Thus, coping effectiveness can range on a continuum from adaptive to maladaptive. There is growing evidence that adaptive coping enhances development and functional performance (Kennedy, 1984; Larson, 1984; Zeitlin, 1985). The more effectively a child copes, the more effectively a child learns. Adaptive coping generates a sense of mastery that is usually reflected in subsequent coping efforts. Maladaptive coping interferes with productive interaction with the environment and therefore hinders learning. Over time, maladaptive coping leads to a sense of incompetence and expectations of failure.

Coping behavior patterns are the repertoire of learned behaviors the child uses to manage the routines, opportunities, challenges, and frustrations encountered in daily living. These behavior patterns are an inner resource that reflects the integration of specific developmental skills to achieve a functional outcome. The patterns become increasingly varied and sophisticated with growth and development. One way of classifying early coping patterns is to cluster them in three categories: sensorimotor, reactive, and self-initiated behaviors. While these categories assist in observing and describing coping behavior, they are not mutually exclusive. The child may use a combination of these behavior patterns in a given situation.

Sensorimotor behavior patterns reflect the child's organization of internal bodily functions and the integration of sensory and motor processes. They include self-regulation, adaptive responses to a variety of sensory stimuli, and the organized use of the sensory and motor systems. These sensorimotor behavior patterns reflect such factors as the organization of state and arousal, the ability to be consoled, self-comforting behaviors, response to the intensity and complexity of sensory stimuli, and the quality of motor control.

Reactive behavior patterns are used to respond to external demands of the physical and social environments. Sample reactive behavior patterns include the ability to accept warmth and support from familiar persons, to react to the feelings and moods of others, to adapt to changes in the environment, and to bounce back after stressful situations.

Self-initiated behavior patterns are autonomously generated, self-directed behaviors used to meet personal needs and to interact with objects and people. Whereas reactive behaviors are closely contingent on environmental cues, self-initiated behaviors are more spontaneous and self-motivated. Sample self-initiated behavior patterns include the ability to explore the environment independently, to initiate action to communicate a need, to apply previously acquired behaviors to new situations, and to change one's behavior when necessary to solve a problem or achieve a goal.

Children who are disabled frequently have fewer resources for developing adaptive coping patterns than their more typical peers. A handicapping condition may interfere with the acquisition of both the developmental skills and adaptive behaviors necessary to cope successfully. However, the presence of a handicapping condition such as spina bifida does not necessarily imply that a child is an ineffective coper. Rather, it suggests a higher degree of vulnerability to the stresses of daily living (Lorch, 1981; Yeargan, 1982; Zeitlin, 1981b). Specific variables such as intelligence, language, temperament and social skills contribute to coping behaviors, but coping, as an integrative process, is different and more comprehensive than any single variable. Therefore, it is important for the preschool team to assesses the coping behavior patterns of the child and to understand how these behaviors influence the child's learning. Many children will need assistance in acquiring more effective management strategies in order to cope adaptively with the demands of the classroom, home, and community.

Determining the Child's Individual Program

In planning an individual educational and therapeutic program for a child, the assessment by the interdisciplinary team addresses the child's developmental capabilities, coping behaviors, and the environmental resources that influence the child's functional performance. A variety of developmental assessment instruments are available to evaluate the child's strengths and weaknesses in such areas as movement, communication, cognition, and personal-social skills. *The Coping Inventory* (Zeitlin, 1985) is a helpful instrument for assessing the behavior patterns that are most relevant to the adaptive coping of children 3 years of age and over. The *Early Coping Inventory* (Zeitlin, Williamson, & Szczepanski, 1986) assesses the coping behavior of children under 3 years of age. The goal of assessment is to gain information about what the child can do (content and skills) and how the child does it (coping process).

Once the child's level of functioning has been determined, the interdisciplinary team decides which factors facilitate the child's learning and which interfere with the learning process. This step is essential in helping the team identify the child's preferred learning style and the strengths the child brings to the learning situation. At the same time, the factors or problems that interfere with learning are analyzed to identify priorities for intervention. Team discussion contributes to the design of goals, objectives, and intervention strategies related to both the expansion of developmental skills and the acquisition of behavior patterns needed by the child for more effective coping. It also prevents fragmentation of the child's program along isolated disciplinary lines.

The following decision-making questions assist an interdisciplinary team to identify the most salient issues that need to be addressed in developing an individual program for a child:

1. What are the primary concerns of the parents?
2. What are the major developmental and coping-related needs of the child?
3. What are the factors facilitating and inhibiting learning?

4. What behaviors and environmental factors that interfere with the child's learning can be changed at the present time?
5. What intervention would have the greatest influence for increasing the child's adaptive coping and functional competence during daily activity?

DESIGNING OPPORTUNITIES TO PROMOTE LEARNING

Since the preschool environment is designed around the child's comprehensive needs and the intervention program is based on his or her developmental rate, the child becomes the center of the learning process. The educational relationship is therefore viewed as one of activity by the child and guidance by the adult. This child-centered perspective is crucial, since handicapped children may tend to become overly dependent on relationships that are initiated and directed by adults. The preschool program encourages independent problem solving, both individually and through social interaction with peers. This section discusses strategies for designing the classroom environment and activities in ways that will promote optimal learning.

The Physical Environment

To achieve a child-centered environment, it is important to structure the physical setting in such a way that it fosters learning and independence. This need is particularly relevant to those children who have major problems in mobility, attention, and perceptual processing. Furniture should be child height, with pictures, posters, and bulletin boards at the eye level of the children. Decoration should be simple and aesthetically pleasing, with materials readily accessible. A close-weave, low-nap carpeting on the floor helps prevent slipping. Areas of the classroom should be well defined according to functional use so as to enhance a sense of order. For example, specific activities should be allocated to different areas, and shelves should be designed to store particular toys. The children will then learn where to go to become involved in certain activities, and where educational materials are located and should be returned after use.

Special attention should be given to the environmental factors that can foster or inhibit optimal engagement in learning. The following questions may help to identify why a child is having difficulty in attending to and completing a task:

1. Is the child in a stable position that allows the hands to be available for manipulative activities?
2. Are there auditory distractions that interfere with performance, such as extraneous noise from the street or hallway?
3. Are there visual distractions, such as cluttered walls or work surfaces?
4. Are the instructional materials visually confusing or overly complex?

5. Is the lighting in the classroom appropriate to prevent glare?
6. Does the child have difficulty working in the center of the room or at a table with other children?
7. Does the physical environment allow ample room for free mobility by the motor-handicapped child?

Establishing a Daily Routine

A daily routine in the classroom helps children understand time and order. They learn what is expected of them and become able to predict what comes next. This atmosphere enhances a sense of security and control. A consistent sequence of events, such as circle time, work periods, free play, and snack time, facilitates the development of internal organization (the ability to self-direct one's personal activity).

Once the children become familiar with the predictable sequence of classroom events, modifications in the routine can be gradually introduced to encourage flexibility and adaptive coping. This step can be accomplished by providing small changes in the routine (e.g., circle time in a different location in the classroom) or altering the routine entirely (e.g., a birthday or holiday party). In this way, the children learn to appreciate the necessity of change, to adapt to change, and to evolve alternative courses of action to meet disruptions in routine. For instance, when rain prevents playing outdoors, the children can be encouraged to choose gross motor games appropriate for the classroom or gym. Such free-choice experiences are significant for children who may be accustomed to having adults schedule all their daily activities.

Structuring Educational Experiences

Preschool children need to develop self-initiated coping behaviors so that they can be active participants in the learning process. It is a skillful teacher who can provide a learning environment that entices a child to become engaged in purposeful activity. The careful design of the classroom space and materials is a critical first step in reaching such a goal. Another important factor is the shifting role of the teacher from active facilitator to observer. At times, practitioners must direct the child's efforts so that learning is experienced as a positive event. At other times, adults need to assume an observational role to give the child an opportunity for free choice, independent exploration, and incidental learning. Some children with myelomeningocele may require a longer time to attempt and complete tasks than their nonhandicapped peers. The following are suggestions for structuring educational experiences in a way that will facilitate learning:

1. The adult should present activities that are designed to meet individual learning needs, are adapted for specific motor disabilities, and are sequenced through the developmental hierarchy of skill acquisition. There should be sufficient familiarity with the task so that the child

recognizes elements from previous experiences, and sufficient unfamiliarity to create a challenge for learning. Control of error can be structured within the materials so that the child can correct mistakes and proceed at an individual pace.

2. Verbal directions that are initially simple and accompanied by demonstration should be provided. Verbal cues should help the child focus on relevant aspects of the task so that the child can solve problems independently. Gradually, the complexity of the verbal directions can be increased and less visual demonstration provided.

3. Positive language should be used when instructing the child. For example, instead of saying, "Pay attention and finish the puzzle," one can say, "You can put the puzzle pieces back in the puzzle" or "I like the way you took the pieces out; now it is time to put them back in."

4. The adult must know the child's capabilities in all developmental areas. In this way, one can be clear about expectations for performance, and comfortable, realistic limits can be set. The child is more likely to experience success when demands match capabilities; and as the child experiences success, conflicts and power struggles are avoided.

5. Concepts and activities should be presented on a regular, systematic basis to reinforce learning. Activities presented in random sequence are not as meaningful for the child and may be disorganizing. Later, concepts should be repeated in a variety of contexts in order to encourage generalization.

6. The adult should help the child identify the start and finish of a specific task so that the child is aware of what needs to be done to complete it. If attention to the activity is poor, one can assist the child to finish it in the way that will best enable the child to experience the feeling of success associated with task completion. Some children may then require guidance in the transition to the next activity.

7. Novelty can be added to the task if the child's attention span is short. For example, the child may be attempting to sort objects by shape, such as circles and squares. Novelty can be introduced by placing the sorted circles in a bucket and the sorted squares in a box.

8. The child's physical status should be monitored with regard to such factors as hunger and fatigue, which influence the ability to learn. Because of motor and learning difficulties, the child with spina bifida may tire more rapidly than other children. The adult should vary activities so as to alternate standing, sitting at a table, and playing on the floor. One should be alert, however, that the child does not habitually use fatigue as an excuse to avoid attempting or completing work.

9. Structured tasks should be followed with unstructured, free-choice activities in order to give the child a sense of control over the learning process.

10. The practitioner should maintain an active communication with the parents by using a notebook which accompanies the child to school and home each day. Professionals can suggest activities in the home that reinforce classroom learning; parents can comment on how the activities succeeded, ask questions, or offer suggestions for further activities. This dialogue is particularly important for assisting children whose skills in communication are limited. Events at home and school are thus shared between the adults so that they can respond consistently to the child's behavior and concerns.

Group Activities

Children with spina bifida may initially find group situations difficult. They may be distracted by the other children and unable to focus on either the teacher or the presented material. However, circle time and other group activities provide excellent opportunities to develop attending behavior. Activities to foster attention include singing songs that are accompanied by gestures, listening for one's name and the names of other children, and focusing on objects during "Show and Tell." The child with attention problems can sit next to the teacher or aide in order to receive verbal cuing or physical prompting (e.g., the adult places his or her hand on the child's knee to regain attention or repositions the child for greater comfort). The teacher can alter the tone of the voice or ring a bell (arousal techniques) to give emphasis to certain activities.

Short, simple stories can be presented, with the children answering questions or retelling the story afterward. Gradually, the stories can be expanded in length. Preschool children often attend intermittently to speech by adults. Expectations for attending to the entire story or conversation can be increased over time. Listening and waiting for one's turn is also an important aspect of the child's participation in group situations.

Group activities offer opportunities to develop awareness of the feelings of others, to learn to help other children, and in general to learn how to be a friend. It is useful for the teacher to label the moods and reactions of the children in order to increase their understanding of the feelings of their peers. In addition, the teacher can encourage the children to assist one another in completing group activities. For example, the child with poor mobility can learn to ask a classmate to retrieve a ball that has rolled away. Emphasis on peer interaction reduces over-reliance on adults for assistance and direction.

ENCOURAGING INDEPENDENCE IN THE CLASSROOM

In the classroom setting, children are encouraged to be as independent as possible. The teacher's approach is modified only as is necessary to meet particular needs of the child.

Fostering Self-Care Skills

When it is determined that the child requires special intervention to develop skills in self-care, instruction can be altered in the following ways:

1. Teaching the task in small, achievable steps
2. Adapting demonstrations and verbal instructions to the particular child
3. Allowing adequate time for the child to complete the task
4. Providing alternative methods for accomplishing the activity (e.g., introducing different techniques for managing a coat)
5. Altering the child's physical position to facilitate the task (e.g., having the child wash his or her hands while sitting at the sink if standing balance is poor)
6. Altering the criteria for success when indicated

The young preschool child may have had little opportunity to develop self-help skills or may enter preschool with expectations that adults or peers will meet his or her self-care needs. It is important for the teacher to create an atmosphere in which necessary assistance is provided while independence is simultaneously fostered. The number of tasks that are automatically accomplished for the child by others should be kept to a minimum. An initial step toward self-sufficiency may be establishing the child's responsibility to communicate a need for help through gesture or verbal request.

Chapter 8 discusses self-care activities in detail. However, the following discussion provides some practical suggestions for managing dressing and toileting activities in the classroom setting.

Dressing   Several factors influence the child's ability to perform dressing tasks in the classroom. They include physical factors (e.g., trunk balance, strength and coordination of the arms, and quality of sensation) as well as the presence of braces and special shoes. Unless the child is an independent ambulator with good balance, removal and replacement of outer garments can most successfully be accomplished in a chair or sitting on the floor. The commonly used "over the head" method may be the easiest technique for achieving independence in donning coats and jackets. Manipulating buttons and other fasteners may be difficult for the preschool child with delayed development of fine motor control. These children may require a variety of preparatory experiences before buttoning is a realistic expectation (see Chapter 6).

Toileting   Classroom personnel need to be aware of the specific procedures for bowel and bladder management used with each child. This information can usually be obtained from the parents or health care professionals. It is important to know whether the child has achieved any control of bowel or bladder function and the nature of the established toileting schedule. Depending on the lesion level, each child will have different degrees of control and requirements for assistance.

By the time they reach preschool age, most children with spina bifida are aware that their toileting needs are different from those of other children. This is particularly true when the child must be diapered or when catheterization is used. The child may be embarrassed by having to wear a diaper or fearful of having accidents in the presence of peers. Sensitivity to the child's feelings is necessary in order to promote a positive self-image. One adult should have primary responsibility to assist with the child's toileting. Consistency is important for establishing a routine and making the child more comfortable with the situation. The child's right to privacy can be honored by diapering the child in the bathroom or in a private changing room. Children who use a toilet may require grab bars for safe transfers and security in sitting.

Although bowel and bladder control may be absent, strategies should be implemented early to develop independent management. Critical factors include the child's physical capabilities, level of judgment, and ability to attend to and sequence the task. Thus, a child with attention deficits may need specific verbal instruction and supervision for success. The child can begin to participate in the diapering process in the following ways:

1. Indicate the need for a diaper change
2. Assist in pulling the pants down, and, if worn, help in removing the long-leg braces
3. Unfasten the soiled diaper
4. Refasten the clean diaper after it is properly positioned
5. Assist in pulling up the pants

Special care is needed to ensure that the child can safely wash his or her hands at the sink after toileting. If the child ambulates with crutches, it may be sufficient to use one crutch for balance while washing and drying. Other children will need to sit on a chair by the sink during this activity.

Mobility

Teachers and other practitioners should be knowledgeable regarding the use, care, and management of braces, crutches, and wheelchairs. A child with long-leg braces may initially require assistance in locking and unlocking hip and knee joints; but development of this skill can be encouraged as early as possible and is generally a realistic expectation during the preschool years.

The child will require instruction on proper storage of crutches or the walker when not in use. Generally, crutches are stored within arm's reach of the child, but in such a way as not to be a hazard to the other children—that is, the crutches should be placed so that classmates do not trip over them. Classmates benefit from instruction in the use of crutches and the need for them to be kept in a place where the child with spina bifida can reach them. In a situation where a child is not able to retrieve crutches, the child can be assigned a peer helper to obtain them. Generally, when there is need for assistance, peers should be utilized as much as possible. This practice not only decreases the child's dependence on adults but also fosters social interaction with peers.

Some children may require help transferring in and out of regular chairs (see Chapter 8). This process is facilitated by selecting a chair of appropriate height and obtaining guidance from the therapist as to specific handling procedures for proper transferring and positioning. In most cases, the child will require assistance from an adult to move the chair up to the table. Assistance is also often needed by children when transferring in and out of a wheelchair.

Independence in carrying such items as toys and educational materials is encouraged by use of a small basket or satchel that can be attached to the walker or wheelchair. Play shopping carts can be employed in the classroom and in some cases may serve as a substitute for crutches for ambulating short distances. For example, a push cart can be utilized after activities to transport materials back to shelves. Child-size back packs may be helpful when commuting to and from school.

GROSS MOTOR ACTIVITIES IN THE CLASSROOM

Gross motor activities are an important component of a comprehensive preschool curriculum. They provide the child with movement experiences and the opportunity for social interaction with peers in a play setting. Initially, the teacher can seek assistance in program planning by consulting with other professionals to determine the extent to which a particular child can participate in gross motor tasks. If the child is receiving therapy services, a classroom visit from the physical or occupational therapist can assist in designing a program in which the child can be an active participant. Familiarity with the needs of the child will facilitate confidence in handling him or her and reduce fear about the child getting hurt during gross motor activity. The ability to manage braces, wheelchairs, and other special equipment is an essential skill for all classroom personnel.

Movement experiences are selected in accordance with the child's ability and modified according to the disability. In general, children with spina bifida are able to participate in many age-appropriate motor activities, with some modification. Cooperative games can be selected to provide the child with successful experiences with peers.

Braces should not be viewed as a deterrent to engaging in physical activity. Such appliances assist the child to develop his or her maximal motor potential. Depending on the weight of the braces, a child may require additional time to complete a task. If crutches or walkers are used, modification of the speed requirements is necessary for walking and running activities. Generally, it is important that the child participate in gross motor games both in and out of the braces, depending on the specific task. Precautions should be taken to avoid skin abrasions on the buttocks and legs in children whose sensitivity to pain and touch is absent or diminished.

For some children, the primary means of independent mobility is the wheelchair. Frequently, the preschool child is just learning how to manage the wheelchair in daily activities. By collaborating with the physical or occupational therapist, the teacher can create recreational games that will promote independence in propelling the wheelchair.

Educators have a wide variety of creative ideas for planning and implementing gross motor activities. Teachers are encouraged to use these ideas to develop their own repertoire of activities based on their classroom curricula and the needs of the child with spina bifida. The following group activities can be structured to accommodate children with a diversity of physical abilities.

Rolling Activities

Rolling can occur on a variety of surfaces, up or down an inclined ramp, or under a "bridge" made of rope. Sensory awareness can be enhanced by having rolling take place with the child wrapped in a sheet or blanket, inside a pillow case, or inside a carpeted barrel. Novelty can be added to the activity by having the child roll to a specific destination to retrieve an object or roll into a tower of cardboard boxes in order to knock it over. The children can also be asked to roll while imitating different objects—such as rolling like a pencil with arms held overhead or rolling like a ball with arms crossed and close to the chest.

Crawling Activities

Most children with myelomeningocele can belly crawl (using primarily the elbows for propulsion), and many are capable of a modified crawl on all four extremities. Obstacle courses can be created in which the child maneuvers over, under, up, down, and through objects in the environment. Other games in the prone or all-fours position include pushing balls of varied sizes to peers in a circle or tossing them at a target. Tunnels, frequently found in the preschool classroom, offer an opportunity for a variety of creative gross motor games in which crawling can readily be incorporated.

Scooter Board Games

Preschool children enjoy games with scooter boards, which are excellent for developing strength and bilateral coordination of the arms. The children can take turns on the scooters, or they can participate in group activities if sufficient equipment is available. In the prone position on the scooter boards, they can move through an obstacle course. Care is needed to ensure that the child's legs do not drag on the floor. If the child cannot propel the scooter with the arms, he or she can be pulled while holding on to a hoop or rope. The following suggestions may be helpful in identifying ways to use a scooter board:

1. The adult can tie a rope between two points and have the children pull themselves along the rope in a hand-over-hand fashion while lying in the prone or supine position on the scooter.

2. The adult can place cardboard boxes in a line and have the children knock them down and out of the way as they proceed in a forward progression.
3. The adult can set up cardboard boxes in a line and have the children negotiate around the boxes without touching them.
4. The adult can use tape or chalk to mark a curved "road" on the floor and have the children stay on the "road" as they propel the scooters.
5. The children can ride down an inclined ramp to provide experience with fast movement through space.
6. The children can play "Follow the Leader" on scooter boards.

Circle Games in the Sitting Position

The child with myelomeningocele can participate in circle games when the children are seated on the floor or in chairs. When trunk control is poor and safe independent sitting has not yet been achieved, a floor seat can be used. For these children, external support is necessary in order to free the arms to engage in the activity. In many cases, a child has better control when seated in an adapted regular chair than on the floor.

The following group activities foster trunk control, coordinated use of the arms, perceptual skills, and social interaction:

1. Ball games can take the form of passing the ball to the right or left, passing it overhead, tossing or bouncing it to peers, or throwing it at a target in the center of the circle. The activity can be graded by using balls of different sizes or bean bags of varying weight. Catching balloons provides the children with additional time to prepare and react, since balloons move more slowly than balls.
2. The children can hold onto a large sheet with both hands, and move the sheet up and down in response to the adult's verbal directions to move it "slow" or "fast." Balloons or foam balls can be placed in the center of the sheet and bounced up and down as the sheet is shaken, to make "popcorn."
3. The children can play "Simon Says" using the arms. Movement patterns can be graded by initially presenting bilateral, symmetrical movements in which both arms perform the same action. Later, reciprocal movements can be emphasized in which the same action is performed alternately by first one arm and then the other. Finally, the children are able to handle more difficult patterns in which the two arms perform different movements simultaneously (e.g., one hand moves to the head while the other moves to the knee). It is important to introduce actions that require crossing the midline of the body with the arms (e.g., right hand to left ear). These tasks reinforce an awareness of the two sides of the body as a functional unit (bilateral integration). "Simon Says" can be varied by giving the children two differently colored streamers of ribbon. The children imitate movements of the teacher with the streamers.

4. Action songs can easily be performed during circle time. Such songs as "Wheels on the Bus" assist the children to learn timing and rhythm.

Play Equipment

The child who has independent sitting balance with good trunk control can be provided with the opportunity to play on gross motor equipment such as rocking boats or horses, large inflatable shapes, slides, and tunnels. Such experience is also important for the child with poor trunk control, but physical support may be required for safe participation. Climbing equipment is appropriate for children who have achieved independent walking with a minimum of orthopaedic appliances. Play equipment should be checked periodically for splinters and rough edges, as a protective measure.

Motor and Sensory Levels of the Spinal Cord

PRIMARY INNERVATION TO THE MUSCLES

Upper Limb Muscles

C. 3, 4   Trapezius; levator scapulae.

C. 5   Rhomboids; deltoids; supraspinatus; infraspinatus; teres minor; biceps.

C. 6   Serratus anterior; latissimus dorsi; subscapularis; teres major; pectoralis major (clavicular head); biceps; coracobrachialis; brachialis; brachioradialis; supinator; extensor carpi radialis longus.

C. 7   Serratus anterior; latissimus dorsi; pectoralis major (sternal head); pectoralis minor; triceps; pronator teres; flexor carpi radialis; flexor digitorum superficialis; extensor carpi radialis longus; extensor carpi radialis brevis; extensor digitorum; extensor digiti minimi.

C. 8   Pectoralis major (sternal head); pectoralis minor; triceps; flexor digitorum superficialis; flexor digitorum profundus; flexor pollicis longus; pronator quadratus; flexor carpi ulnaris; extensor carpi ulnaris; abductor pollicis longus; extensor pollicis longus; extensor pollicis brevis; extensor indicis; abductor pollicis brevis; flexor pollicis brevis; opponens pollicis.

T. 1   Flexor digitorum profundus; intrinsic muscles of the hand (except abductor pollicis brevis; flexor pollicis brevis; opponens pollicis).

Lower Limb Muscles

L. 1   Psoas major; psoas minor.

L. 2   Psoas major; iliacus; sartorius; gracilis; pectineus; adductor longus; adductor brevis.

L. 3   Quadriceps; adductors (magnus, longus, brevis).

L. 4   Quadriceps; tensor fasciae latae; adductor magnus; obturator externus; tibialis anterior; tibialis posterior.

L. 5   Gluteus medius; gluteus minimus; obturator internus; semimembranosus; semitendinosus; extensor hallucis longus; extensor digitorum longus and peroneus tertius; popliteus.

S. 1   Gluteus maximus; obturator internus; piriformis; biceps femoris; semitendinosus; popliteus; gastrocnemius; soleus; peronei (longus and brevis); extensor digitorum brevis.

S. 2   Piriformis; biceps femoris; gastrocnemius; soleus; flexor digitorum longus; flexor hallucis longus; intrinsic foot muscles.

S. 3   Intrinsic foot muscles (except abductor hallucis; flexor hallucis brevis; flexor digitorum brevis; extensor digitorum brevis).

Joint Movements

Shoulder	Abductors and lateral rotators.	C. 5
	Adductors and medial rotators.	C. 6, 7, 8
Elbow	Flexors.	C. 5, 6
	Extensors.	C. 7, 8
Forearm	Supinators.	C. 6
	Pronators.	C. 7, 8
Wrist	Flexors and extensors.	C. 6, 7
Digits	Long flexors and extensors	C. 7, 8
Hand	Intrinsic muscles.	C. 8, T. 1
Hip	Flexors, adductors, medial rotators.	L. 1, 2, 3
	Extensors, abductors, lateral rotators.	L. 5, S. 1
Knee	Extensors.	L. 3, 4
	Flexors.	L. 5, S. 1
Ankle	Dorsiflexors.	L. 4, 5
	Plantar flexors.	S. 1, 2
Foot	Invertors.	L. 4, 5
	Evertors.	L. 5, S. 1

CUTANEOUS DISTRIBUTION OF SPINAL NERVES

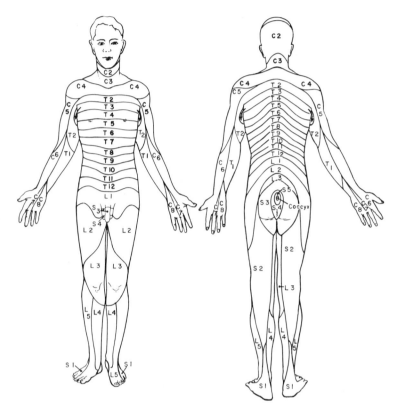

Source: Barr, M. L., & Kiernan, J. A. (1983). *The human nervous system: A medical viewpoint* (4th ed., p. 79). Hagerstown, MD: Harper & Row; reprinted by permission.

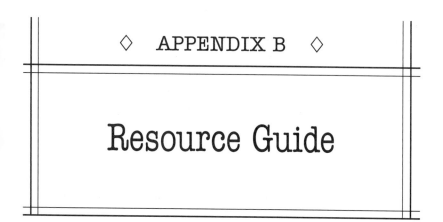

Resource Guide

Accent on Living
Box 700
Bloomington, IL 61701
(309) 378-2961

Source of information for individuals with physical disabilities. Publishes a quarterly magazine that provides news, practical assistance regarding daily living, and listings of products and services for disabled persons.

Consumer Care Products, Inc.
6405 Paradise Land
Sheboygan Falls, WI 53085
(414) 467-3600

Hand-driven tricycle with back support, foot modifications, and vertical handles.

Educational Resource Information Center (ERIC)
ERIC Clearinghouse on Handicapped and Gifted Children
1920 Association Drive
Reston, VA 22091
(703) 620-3660

Computerized information system that can be accessed at any of 800 subscribing libraries across the country. Annotated bibliographies available by subject.

Equipment Shop
Box 33
Bedford, MA 01730
(617) 275-7681

Adapted furniture (e.g., prone standers, corner seats, floor tables), Gymnastik therapy balls, hardware for tricycle modifications, and peg handles for walker adaptations. Distributor of the Cyclone, a hand-powered riding vehicle for children that accommodates for long-leg braces.

Everest and Jennings
3233 East Mission Oaks Boulevard
Camarillo, CA 93010
(800) 235-4661

Manufacturer of wheelchairs and mobility devices, including the Ultralite pediatric wheelchair that is lightweight and adjustable for growth.

Federation for Children with Special Needs
312 Stuart Street
Boston, MA 02116
(617) 482-2915
Agency coordinates federally funded parent information, training, and advocacy centers across the country. Parents can contact the federation for the address of a center nearest to them.

Fred Sammons, Inc.
Box 32
Brookfield, IL 60513
(800) 323-5547
Therapeutic supplies, adapted equipment, and self-help aids for eating, dressing, and hygiene.

Guardian Products
780 Easy Street
Box 549
Simi Valley, CA 93065
(800) 524-1703
Walkers and mobility aids from toddler through adult sizes.

J.A. Preston Corporation
60 Page Road
Clifton, NJ 07012
(800) 631-7277
Therapeutic supplies, adapted equipment, and mobility aids for children and adults. Distributor of Tumble Forms rolls, wedges, and feeder seats of various sizes.

Johnson and Johnson
Baby Products Company
Child Development Products Division
Grandview Road
Skillman, NJ 08558
(800) 526-3967
Toys for infants and toddlers that are based on sound research in child development. A mail order toy program is available.

Modular Medical Corporation
1558 Hutchinson River Parkway East
Bronx, NY 10461
(212) 829-2626
Source for Adapta foam (varying sizes, shapes, and densities) and the latex-like protective coating required for finishing.

National Health Information Clearinghouse
Box 1133
Washington, DC 20013
(800) 336-4797
Information resource for parents and professionals regarding health-related questions.

National Information Center for Handicapped Children and Youth
1555 Wilson Boulevard
Suite 508
Rosslyn, VA 22209
(703) 522-3332

Free information service for professionals and parents of children with handicaps.

Rifton Equipment for the Handicapped
Route 213
Rifton, NY 12471
(914) 658-3141

Manufacturer and distributor of Rifton equipment including sidelyers, prone standers, scooter boards, tricycles, child-size commodes, bath seats, chairs, and tables of various kinds (e.g., easel-style and standing tables). Equipment is well-constructed, durable, and adjustable.

Spina Bifida Association of America
1700 Rockville Pike
Suite 540
Rockville, MD 20852
(800) 621-3141

Major national advocacy organization with chapters located throughout the United States for individuals with spina bifida and their families. Publishes a regular newsletter and has an extensive list of available publications appropriate for parents and professionals. Supports public education, research, and legislation related to spina bifida.

Glossary

Abduction   Movement away from the center line (midline) of the body.

Adduction   Movement toward the center line (midline) of the body.

Alternating strabismus   Imbalance of the eye muscles in which deviation varies alternately from one eye to the other.

Anterior tilt of the pelvis   Forward tilting of the pelvis controlled by muscle action of the hip flexors and low back extensors. A marked anterior tilt of the pelvis results in lumbar hyperextension (lordosis).

Apraxia   Inability to organize and execute unfamiliar (novel) motor acts.

Arnold-Chiari malformation   Abnormal displacement of the medulla (lower portion of the brain stem) and the cerebellum that causes problems in controlling movement.

Asymmetrical tonic neck reflex   Turning of the head to the side that results in an increase in extensor muscle tone on the side the face is turned toward and an increase of flexor tone on the opposite (skull) side. Seen in normal motor development until approximately 4 months of age when it becomes integrated.

Bear-walk position   Body weight is supported on the hands and feet with the hips flexed and knees extended.

Bilateral   Involving two sides of the body (e.g., reaching with both hands).

Bilateral integration   Ability of the two sides of the brain to communicate and work harmoniously, resulting in coordinated use of the two sides of the body together.

Binocular vision   Simultaneous use of both eyes together in normal (conjugate) vision.

Body scheme   Inner awareness of one's body parts, the relationship of these parts to the body as a whole, and how the parts move together through space.

Brain stem reflexes   Static, postural reflexes controlled by the brain stem. They are elicited by a change in the position of the head or the body in space and cause a redistribution of muscle tone throughout the body (e.g., asymmetrical tonic neck reflex, tonic labyrinthine reflex).

Bridging   In the supine position, lifting up the buttocks off the support surface so that the hips are extended and the knees are flexed.

Catheter   Tube used to drain urine from the bladder.

Cerebrospinal fluid   Clear fluid surrounding the brain and spinal cord that acts as a shock absorber to protect these internal structures.

Cocktail party syndrome   Hyperverbal speech reflecting a semantic-pragmatic language problem. Characterized by a good ability to use language forms (sentences and grammatical structure) but difficulty in content (meaning) and use (functions and purpose) of language.

Contracture   Limitation in the range of motion of a joint.

Convergence   Ability to direct both eyes simultaneously inward to focus on a near point or an approaching object. The closer the object, the greater the degree of convergence required to focus.

Coping   Active process of using one's resources to meet personal needs and to adapt to the demands of the environment in ways that maintain or enhance feelings of well-being.

Coping behaviors   Repertoire of learned behaviors the child uses to manage routines, opportunities, challenges, and frustrations encountered in daily living.

Craig-Scott brace   Long-leg brace with a three-point pressure system to maintain the hip and knee in extension and to stabilize the ankle for standing and ambulation with crutches.

Cystitis   Urinary tract infection common in children with spina bifida.

Cystogram   X-ray procedure to detect reflux of urine from the bladder into the ureters after the bladder has been filled with radio-opaque fluid.

Cystometrogram   Study of bladder function in which graphic recordings are obtained of muscle contractions of the bladder wall in response to stretch induced by injection of a mild saline solution into the bladder.

Cystoscopic examination   Evaluation of the interior of the bladder by viewing through a cystoscope (a small tube with a lighted end that is inserted into the bladder).

Digital-pronate grasp   Grasp pattern in which the crayon or utensil is held with the distal portion of the fingers and thumb while the forearm remains pronated (palm turned down).

Dissociation   Refinement of gross patterns of movement into more isolated, discrete motions of the body part.

Dorsiflexion   Movement at the talocalcaneal (upper ankle) joint resulting in the foot pointing up.

Dynamic tripod grasp   Mature, three-point grasp of a crayon or pencil in which the wrist is slightly extended, the thumb opposes the distal ends of the index and middle fingers, and the ring and little fingers are flexed to provide a supportive arch for the hand. This grasp employs only fine movements of the fingers to direct the pencil.

Equilibrium reactions   Automatic postural reactions elicited by stimulation of the labyrinths in the inner ear when the center of gravity is changed through movement of the support surface or the body. These reactions may include subtle changes in muscle tone or obvious movements of the head, trunk, and limbs to restore balance.

Esotropia   Deviation of the eye inward due to a muscle imbalance.

Exotropia   Deviation of the eye outward due to a muscle imbalance.

Extension   Straightening of a joint. A marked degree of extension is called hyperextension (e.g., neck or trunk hyperextension).

Eye-hand coordination   Controlled use of the upper extremities for visually directed reach and manipulation.

Fencing position   Posture resulting from the influence of the asymmetrical tonic neck reflex.

Figure-ground perception   Ability to focus on relevant details in the visual environment by distinguishing foreground from background.

Flexion   Bending of a joint.

Froglike posture   Excessive hip flexion, abduction, and external rotation.

Gestural imitation   Ability to copy the gestures and actions of others.

Glenohumeral joint   Shoulder joint formed by the glenoid fossa of the scapula and the head of the humerus.

Gluteal muscles   Group of three muscles that form the contour of the buttock originating at the pelvis and inserting on the femur (thigh bone). These muscles are primarily responsible for extending the hip but also contribute to movements of abduction, adduction, and rotation at the hip joint.

Hemispheric specialization   Tendency of the two hemispheres of the brain to develop major responsibility for processing and directing particular functions (e.g., language, spatial perception).

Hydrocephalus   Excessive accumulation of cerebrospinal fluid in the ventricles of the brain due to blocked fluid circulation, resulting in compression of the brain and eventually enlargement of the head.

Hyperopia   "Farsightedness" or difficulty seeing near objects. A refractive error in which light rays reach the retina before coming to a proper focus.

Hypertonicity   Abnormal increase in muscle tone. Also referred to as spasticity.

Intravenous pyelogram (IVP)   X-ray procedure that provides information on the anatomy of the ureters and the function of the kidneys.

Kinesthesia   Awareness of joint motion.

Kyphosis   Exaggeration of the posterior convexity of the thoracic spine resulting in a "hunchback" posture.

Labyrinths   Structure in the inner ear that contains the sensory receptors of the vestibular system (the semicircular canals that detect changes in head position and the otoliths that respond to the pull of gravity).

Lateral flexion   Bending of the joint to the side, as in lateral flexion of the neck or the trunk.

Lateral prehension   Grasp of an object between the thumb and the side of the index finger. Sometimes referred to as a scissor grasp or an inferior pincer grasp.

Lofstrand crutches   Forearm crutches.

Long sitting   Sitting position with legs straight out in front of the body.

Lordosis   Anterior convexity of the lumbar spine. Commonly referred to as a swayback posture when the lordosis is increased.

Means-end skill   Ability to use problem solving to achieve an end or reach a goal.

Meningocele   Protrusion of the protective covering of the spinal cord (the meninges) through an opening in the spinal column to form a sac. If the spinal cord and nerves remain intact, there tends to be no neurological deficit after surgical removal of the sac.

Moro reflex Automatic reaction causing extension and abduction of the arms, frequently followed by flexion and adduction across the body. Usually elicited by gently dropping the infant's head backward when he or she is held in a partially upright position. Typically observed in normal infants from birth to 4–6 months of age.

Muscle tone Underlying, normal tension in the muscle that is due to a low-grade contraction or the elasticity of the muscle fibers themselves. It provides a readiness for the muscles to engage in voluntary movement.

Myelodysplasia Defective formation of the spinal cord.

Myelomeningocele Protrusion of the meninges and a portion of the spinal cord through an opening in the spine to form a sac. The spinal cord and nerves are usually damaged, resulting in a neurological deficit.

Myopia "Nearsightedness" or difficulty with distance vision. A refractive error in which light rays focus in front of, rather than on, the retina.

Neat pincer grasp Fine prehension of an object between the tip of the thumb and the tip of the forefinger. Also referred to as a fine pincer grasp or fingertip prehension.

Neurogenic bladder Deficiency in the nerve supply to the bladder resulting in an inability to void in a controlled and voluntary manner.

Nystagmus Involuntary jerking movements of the eyes.

Object permanence Awareness that objects have an independent existence even when they are not seen.

Opisthotonus Marked arching of the body into extension due to spastic extensor muscles.

Opposition Motion of the thumb that allows it to approximate the ends of the fingers for pinch and manipulation of objects.

Orthoses Orthopaedic appliances such as shoe inserts, splints, and braces.

Osteoporosis Increased porosity and softening of a bone that can predispose it to fractures.

Palmar grasp Gross grasp pattern in which the fingers are used to press an object against the palm.

Palmar-supinate grasp Grasp pattern typically used for crayons and utensils, combining a palmar grasp (fisted hand) and supination of the forearm to a midposition.

Parachute reaction Automatic thrust of the arms forward when the infant is quickly lowered head down in a vertical position toward a supporting surface.

Parapodium Standing device that provides maximal support to the trunk and legs in order to maintain an independent upright posture without hand support.

Pincer grasp Grasp of an object between the thumb and the index finger.

Plantarflexion Movement at the talocalcaneal (upper ankle) joint resulting in the foot pointing down.

Play schemes Use of a variety of actions and strategies when playing with objects.

Posterior tilt of the pelvis Backward tilting of the pelvis controlled by the action of the abdominal and hip extensor muscles. A posterior tilt of the pelvis results in rounding of the lumbar spine (low back).

Proprioceptors Sensory receptors in the muscles, tendons, and joints that provide an appreciation of the position of body parts during movement and at rest.

Protective extension Automatic thrust of an upper or lower extremity away from the body to prevent falling.

Quadruped   All-fours position assumed on hands and knees, as in crawling.

Radial-digital grasp   Grasp pattern in which an object is held between the thumb and the ends of the fingers.

Radial-palmar grasp   Grasp pattern in which an object is pressed by the fingers against the palm and the base of the thumb.

Raking grasp   Scraping or scratching the hand and fingers against a surface in an attempt to retrieve an object.

Reciprocating hip extension brace   Long-leg brace with a cable mechanism to decrease the tendency toward hip flexion when standing and walking. Designed to enhance a reciprocal gait pattern.

Righting reactions   Automatic postural reactions that maintain an upright position of the head in space and restore symmetrical alignment of the head and trunk.

Ring sitting   Sitting position with hips flexed and abducted forming a "ring" on the floor that provides a wide base of support.

Rotation   Twisting movements (e.g., the turning in and turning out of a limb or twisting the trunk toward the right or the left).

Scapula   Shoulder blade.

Scoliosis   Lateral bend or side-to-side curvature of the spine that may be accompanied by varying degrees of abnormal rotation of the spinal column.

Sensory integration   Normal processing of the brain that enables one to receive and interpret sensory information from the body and the environment in order to make purposeful, adaptive responses.

Shift of gaze   Ability to change visual fixation from one object to another.

Short sitting   Sitting position assumed on a chair with hips, knees, and ankles at 90° of flexion.

Shunt   Flexible tube surgically inserted from the ventricles to the heart (ventriculo-atrial shunt) or the abdominal cavity (ventriculoperitoneal shunt) to drain excess cerebrospinal fluid from the brain.

Somatosensory perception   Integration and interpretation of vestibular, tactile, and proprioceptive sensation. It contributes to the development of body scheme and motor planning.

Spatial relationships   Ability to appreciate the orientation of objects and sounds in space, and their relationship to the self and to each other.

Spina bifida   Congenital malformation of the spine characterized by failure of the vertebrae to fuse or close. Commonly referred to as a neural tube defect.

Spina bifida cystica   Generic term referring to both meningocele and myelomeningocele.

Spina bifida occulta   Abnormal opening in the spine due to failure of the back arches of the vertebrae to fuse. The spinal cord and spinal nerves are typically not damaged, and neurological function remains intact.

Standing brace   Prefabricated brace providing maximal support to the trunk and legs to allow for early standing.

Static tripod grasp   Three-point grasp of a crayon or utensil involving the proximal aspect of the thumb and the index and middle fingers. Movement occurs primarily at the wrist with limited motion of the fingers.

Stereognosis   Ability to identify objects solely by touch.

Strabismus   Failure of the eyes to direct their gaze simultaneously at the same object due to muscular imbalance.

Swing-through gait   Ambulation pattern with crutches in which the legs swing forward together beyond the placement of the crutch tips.

Swing-to gait   Ambulation pattern with crutches in which the legs swing forward together to the placement of the crutch tips.

Symbolic play   Play behavior that is characterized by pretending and using objects and actions to represent something else.

Tonic labyrinthine reflex   A brain stem–level reflex triggered by the labyrinths in the inner ear that results in increased extensor muscle tone in the supine position and flexor tone in the prone position.

Ulnar deviation   Bending of the wrists outward in the direction of the little finger.

Ureter   Tube carrying urine from each kidney to the bladder.

Urethra   A single tube transporting urine from the bladder for elimination.

Urinalysis   Laboratory analysis of the urine including a culture to determine the presence of bacteria.

Urinary reflux   Backflow of urine from the bladder into the ureters.

Ventricles   Cavities deep within the brain that secrete cerebrospinal fluid.

Vertebrae   Bones that link together to form the spinal column.

Vestibular system   Sensory system involved with the detection and interpretation of movement sensations arising from changes in the head or body in space and the influence of gravity.

Visual acuity   Ability to see objects and their details. Refers to the clarity of vision.

Visual fixation   Ability to direct the eyes and focus on the same point in space for a period of time.

Visual perception   Ability to interpret and understand what is seen with the eyes.

Visual scanning   Ability to change visual fixation in a linear plane among objects that are presented concurrently.

Visual tracking   Ability to move the eyes in various planes to follow a moving target.

Vocal imitation   Ability to reproduce sounds and words that one hears.

References

Agness, P.J. (1983). *Learning disabilities and the person with spina bifida.* Chicago: Spina Bifida Association of America.

Anderson, E.M. (1973). Cognitive deficits in children with spina bifida and hydrocephalus: A review of the literature. *British Journal of Educational Psychology, 43,* 257.

Anderson, E.M. (1975). *Cognitive and motor deficits in children with spina bifida cystica and hydrocephalus with special reference to writing difficulties.* Unpublished doctoral dissertation, University of London.

Anderson, E.M. (1976). Handwriting difficulties in children with spina bifida and hydrocephalus. *Special Education Forward Trends, 3,* 17–20.

Anderson, E.M., & Spain, B. (1977). *The child with spina bifida.* London: Methuen.

Ayres, A.J. (1979). *Sensory integration and the child.* Los Angeles: Western Psychological Services.

Badell-Ribera, A. (1985). Myelodysplasia. In G.E. Molnar (Ed.), *Pediatric rehabilitation.* Baltimore: Williams & Wilkins.

Balzer-Martin, L.A. (1980). A study to determine the relationships existing between sensory integrative functioning and performance IQ in children with myelomeningocele (Doctoral dissertation, American University, 1980). *Dissertation Abstracts International, 41* (10-A), 4356.

Barden, G.A., Meyer, L.C., & Stelling, F.H. (1975). Myelodysplastics: Fate of those followed for twenty years or more. *Journal of Bone and Joint Surgery, 57A,* 643–647.

Barr, M.L., & Kiernan, J.A. (1983). *The human nervous system: A medical viewpoint* (4th ed.). Hagerstown, MD: Harper & Row.

Bates, E., Benigni, L., Bretherton, I., Camaioni, L., & Volterra, V. (1979). *The emergence of symbols: Cognition and communication in infancy.* New York: Academic Press.

Bergen, A.F., & Colangelo, C. (1985). *Positioning the client with C.N.S. deficits: The wheelchair and other adapted equipment* (2nd ed.). Valhalla, NY: Valhalla Rehabilitation Publications.

Berns, J.H. (1980). Grandparents of handicapped children. *Social Work, 25,* 238–239.

Blackwell, K., Britz, H., Jans, C., Rock, K., & Vedovatti, P. (1981). Information for visual programming with physically multihandicapped students. In R. York, W.K. Schofield, Jr., & D.J. Donder (Eds.), *Organizing and implementing services for students with severe and multiple handicaps.* Springfield: Illinois State Board of Education.

Blank, M., Rose, S.R., & Berlin, L.J. (1978). *The language of learning*. New York: Grune & Stratton.

Bleck, E.E. (1975). Myelomeningocele, meningocele, spina bifida. In E.E. Bleck & D.A. Nagel (Eds.), *Physically handicapped children: A medical atlas for teachers*. New York: Grune & Stratton.

Bloom, L., & Lahey, M. (1978). *Language development and language disorders*. New York: John Wiley & Sons.

Bloom, L., Rocissano, L., & Hood, L. (1976). Adult-child discourse: Developmental interaction between information processing and linguistic knowledge. *Cognitive Psychology, 8,* 521–552.

Bly, L. (1983). *The components of normal movement during the first year of life and abnormal motor development*. Chicago: Neuro-Developmental Treatment Association.

Borzyskowski, M. (1984). Management of neuropathic bladder in childhood. *Developmental Medicine and Child Neurology, 26,* 401–404.

Brocklehurst, G. (Ed.). (1976). *Spina bifida for the clinician*. Philadelphia: J.B. Lippincott.

Brown, H.P. (1978). Management of spinal deformity in myelomeningocele. *Orthopedic Clinics of North America, 9,* 391–402.

Brunt, D. (1980). Characteristics of upper limb movements in a sample of meningomyelocele children. *Perceptual and Motor Skills, 51,* 431–437.

Carlson, D., & Stone, D.P. (1982). Teaching clean intermittent catheterization. *Clinical Proceedings: Children's Hospital National Medical Center, 38,* 161–167.

Carroll, N. (1978). Hip instability in children with myelomeningocele. *Orthopedic Clinics of North America, 9,* 403–408.

Carroll, N. (1983). The orthopedic and orthotic management of the spina bifida child. *Clinical Neurosurgery, 30,* 413–435.

Chappell, G. (1982). Alpha-feta protein testing and informed consent. *Clinical Proceedings: Children's Hospital National Medical Center, 38,* 214–216.

Charney, E.B., Weller, S.C., Sutton, L.N., Bruce, D.A., & Schut, L.B. (1985). Management of the newborn with myelomeningocele: Time for a decision-making process. *Pediatrics, 75,* 58–64.

Childs, V. (1977). Physiotherapy for spina bifida. *Physiotherapy, 63,* 218–221.

Cohen, L.B., DeLoache, J.S., & Strauss, M.S. (1979). Infant visual perception. In J.D. Osofsky (Ed.), *Handbook of infant development*. New York: John Wiley & Sons.

Connor, F.P., Williamson, G.G., & Siepp, J.M. (1978). *Program guide for infants and toddlers with neuromotor and other developmental disabilities*. New York: Teachers College Press.

Crowe, C.A., Heuther, C.A., Oppenheimer, S.C., Barth, L.D., Jeffrey, E., & Reinhart, S. (1985). The epidemiology of spina bifida in south-western Ohio: 1970–1979. *Developmental Medicine and Child Neurology, 27,* 176–182.

DeSouza, L.J., & Carroll, N. (1976). Ambulation of the braced myelomeningocele patient. *Journal of Bone and Joint Surgery, 58-A,* 1112–1118.

Dodds, J. (1975). *Hydrocephalic children and visual perception*. Unpublished master's dissertation, University of Sussex, England.

Dore, J. (1975). Holophrases, speech acts and language universals. *Journal of Child Language, 2,* 21–40.

Dore, J. (1978). Variation in preschool children's conversational performance. In K. Nelson (Ed.), *Children's language* (Vol. 1). New York: Gardner Press.

Dunst, C.J. (1981). *Infant learning: A cognitive-linguistic intervention strategy*. Hingham, MA: Teaching Resources.

Erhardt, R.P. (1982). *Developmental hand dysfunction: Theory, assessment, treatment.* Laurel, MD: RAMSCO.

Erikson, E. (1963). *Childhood and society.* New York: W.W. Norton.

Farber, S.D. (1982). *Neurorehabilitation: A multisensory approach.* Philadelphia: W.B. Saunders.

Featherstone, H. (1980). *A difference in the family: Life with a disabled child.* New York: Basic Books.

Feiwell, E., Sakai, D., & Blatt, T. (1978). The effect of hip reduction on function in patients with myelomeningocele: Potential gains and hazards of surgical treatment. *Journal of Bone and Joint Surgery, 60,* 169–173.

Field, T. (1978). The three Rs of infant-adult interactions: Rhythms, repertoires, and responsitivity. *Journal of Pediatric Psychology, 3,* 131–136.

Findley, T.W. (1983). Ambulation and the adolescent with myelomeningocele (Doctoral dissertation, University of Minnesota, 1983). *Dissertation Abstracts International, 44* (9-B), 2704.

Finnie, N. (1975). *Handling the young cerebral palsied child at home* (2nd ed.). New York: E.P. Dutton.

Fiorentino, M.R. (1981). *A basis for sensorimotor development: Normal and abnormal.* Springfield, IL: Charles C Thomas.

Frank, J.D., & Fixsen, J.A. (1980). Spina bifida. *British Journal of Hospital Medicine, 24,* 422–437.

Gallagher, J., Bechman, P., & Cross, A. (1983). Families of handicapped children: Sources of stress and its amelioration. *Exceptional Children, 50,* 10–19.

Germain, C.B. (1973). An ecological perspective in casework practice. *Social Casework, 54,* 323–330.

Gilfoyle, E.M., Grady, A.P., & Moore, J.C. (1981). *Children adapt.* Thorofare, NJ: Charles B. Slack.

Gliedman, J., & Roth, W. (1980). *The unexpected minority: Handicapped children in America.* New York: Harcourt Brace Jovanovich.

Gordon, B. (1972). The superior colliculus of the brain. *Scientific American, 227,* 72–82.

Greer, J.G., & Wethered, C.E. (1984). Learned helplessness: A piece of the burnout puzzle. *Exceptional Children, 50,* 524–530.

Grimm, R. (1976). Hand function and tactile perception in two samples of children with myelomeningocele. *American Journal of Occupational Therapy, 30,* 234–240.

Hall, J.E., & Poitras, B. (1977). The management of kyphosis in patients with myelomeningocele. *Clinical Orthopaedics and Related Research, 128,* 33–40.

Hammock, M.K., & Milhorat, T.H. (1982). Current neurosurgical management of the patient with myelomeningocele. *Clinical Proceedings: Children's Hospital National Medical Center, 38,* 148–155.

Hannigan, K.F. (1979). Teaching intermittent self-catheterization to young children with myelodysplasia. *Developmental Medicine and Child Neurology, 21,* 365–368.

Haynes, U. (1983). *Holistic health care for children with developmental disabilities.* Baltimore: University Park Press.

Hoffman, R.G. (1981). Selective cognitive deficits in myelomeningocele children (Doctoral dissertation, Long Island University, 1981). *Dissertation Abstracts International, 41* (11-B), 4264.

Horn, D.G., Lorch, E.P. Lorch, R.F., Jr., & Culatta, B. (1985). Distractibility and vocabulary deficits in children with spina bifida and hydrocephalus. *Developmental Medicine and Child Neurology, 27,* 713–720.

Hunt, G.M., & Holmes, A.E. (1976). Factors relating to intelligence in treated cases of spina bifida cystica. *The American Journal of Diseases of Children, 130,* 823–827.

Kass, E.J. (1982). Current urological management of the child with myelodysplasia. *Clinical Proceedings: Children's Hospital National Medical Center, 38*, 156–160.

Kazak, A.E., & Marvin, R.S. (1984). Differences, difficulties, and adaptation: Stress and social networks in families with a handicapped child. *Family Relations, 33*, 67–77.

Kearsley, R.B. (1981). Cognitive assessment of the handicapped infant: The need for an alternative approach. *American Journal of Orthopsychiatry, 51*, 43–54.

Kennedy, B. (1984). *The relationship of coping behaviors and attribution of success to effort and school achievement of elementary school children.* Unpublished doctoral dissertation, State University of New York at Albany.

Klaus, M.H. & Kennell, J.H. (1976). *Maternal-infant bonding*.St. Louis: C.V. Mosby.

Knickerbocker, B.M. (1980). *A holistic approach to the treatment of learning disorders.* Thorofare, NJ: Charles B. Slack.

Land, L.C. (1977). A study of the sensory integration of children with myelomeningocele. In R. McLauren (Ed.), *Myelomeningocele.* New York: Grune & Stratton.

Langley, M.B. (1980). *Functional vision inventory for the multiply and severely handicapped.* Chicago: Stoelting.

Larson, J.G. (1984). Relationship between coping behavior and academic achievement in kindergarten children (Doctoral dissertation, Fairleigh Dickinson University, 1984). *Dissertation Abstracts International, 45* (8-A), 2389.

Larson, K.A. (1982). The sensory history of developmentally delayed children with and without tactile defensiveness. *American Journal of Occupational Therapy. 36*, 590–596.

Lauder, C.E., Kanthor, H., Myers, G., & Resnick, J. (1979). Educational placement of children with spina bifida. *Exceptional Children, 45*, 432–437.

Lavelle, N., & Keogh, B. (1980). Expectations and attributions of parents of handicapped children. *New Directions for Exceptional Children, 4*, 1–27.

Lazarus, R., & Folkman, S. (1984). *Stress, appraisal and coping.* New York: Springer.

Leatherman, K.D., & Dickson, R.A. (1978). Congenital kyphosis in myelomeningocele: Vertebral bony resection and posterior spine fusion. *Spine, 3*, 222–226.

Lipsky, D.K. (1985). A parental perspective on stress and coping. *American Journal of Orthopsychiatry, 55*, 614–617.

Lonton, A.P. (1976). Hand preference in children with myelomeningocele and hydrocephalus. *Developmental Medicine and Child Neurology, 18* (Supplement 37), 143–149.

Lorch, N. (1981). Coping behavior in preschool children with cerebral palsy (Doctoral dissertation, Hofstra University, 1981). *Dissertation Abstracts International, 42* (8-B), 3431.

Lucas, E.V. (1980). *Semantic and pragmatic language disorders.* Rockville, MD: Aspen Systems.

Madden, B.K. & Bchir, M.B. (1977). Orthopaedic aspects of spina bifida. *Physiotherapy, 63*, 186–190.

McLone, D.G., Czyzewski, D., Raimondi, A.J., & Sommers, R.C. (1982). Central nervous system infection as a limiting factor in the intelligence of children with myelomeningocele. *Pediatrics, 70*, 338–342.

Menelaus, M.B. (1976). Orthopaedic management of children with myelomeningocele: A plea for realistic goals. *Developmental Medicine and Child Neurology, 18* (Supplement 37), 3–11.

Menelaus, M.B. (1980). Progress in the management of the paralytic hip in my-elomeningocele. *Orthopedic Clinics of North America, 11,* 17–30.

Miller, E., & Sethi, L. (1971). The effect of hydrocephalus on percepton. *Developmental Medicine and Child Neurology, 13,* 77–80.

Miller, J. (Ed.). (1980). *Assessing language production in children* (Vol. 1). Baltimore: University Park Press.

Molnar, G.E. (Ed.). (1985). *Pediatric rehabilitation.* Baltimore: Williams & Wilkins.

Moos, R. (Ed.). (1976). *Human adaptation: Coping with life crises.* Lexington, MA: D.C. Heath.

Morris, S.E. (1977). Assessment and treatment of children with oral-motor dysfunction. In J.M. Wilson (Ed.), *Oral-motor function and dysfunction in children.* Chapel Hill: University of North Carolina, Division of Physical Therapy.

Morris, S.E. (1981). *The normal acquisition of oral feeding skills.* New York: Therapeutic Media.

Murphy, L.B., & Moriarty, A. (1976). *Vulnerability, coping and growth.* New Haven, CT: Yale University Press.

Murphy, M.A. (1982). The family with a handicapped child: A review of the literature. *Developmental and Behavioral Pediatrics, 3,* 73–82.

Myers, G.J. (1984). Myelomeningocele: The medical aspects. *Pediatric Clinics of North America, 31,* 165–175.

Myers, G.J., Cerone, S.B., & Olson, A.L. (1981). *A guide for helping the child with spina bifida.* Springfield, IL: Charles C Thomas.

Nakos, E., & Taylor, S. (1977). *Early development of the child with myelomeningocele: A parent's guide.* Cincinnati: Children's Hospital Medical Center.

Nason, S.S. (1982). Orthopedic management of the child with spina bifida. *Clinical Proceedings: Children's Hospital National Medical Center, 38,* 170–181.

Nelson, V.S., Saffer, A.M., Kling, T.F. & Lewinter, R. (1984). Upper extremity dysfunction in myelodysplastic children. *Developmental Medicine and Child Neurology, 26,* 251–252.

Okamoto, G.A., Sousa, J., Telzrow, R.W., Holm, R.A., McCartin, R., & Shurtleff, D.B. (1984). Toileting skills in children with myelomeningocele: Rates of learning. *Archives of Physical Medicine and Rehabilitation, 65,* 182–185.

Olsen, D., & McCubbin, H. (1983). *Families: What makes them work.* Beverly Hills: Sage Publications.

Peterson, R., & Lippa, S.B. (1978). Life cycle crises encountered by families of developmentally disabled children: Implications and recommendations for practice. *Proceedings of the 102nd Annual Meeting of the American Association on Mental Deficiency.*

Piaget, J. (1952). *The origins of intelligence in children.* New York: International Universities Press.

Piggott, H. (1980). The natural history of scoliosis in myelodysplasia. *Journal of Bone and Joint Surgery, 62,* 54–58.

Pinyerd, B.J. (1983). Siblings of children with myelomeningocele: Examining their perceptions. *Maternal-Child Nursing Journal, 12,* 61–70.

Prigatano, G.P., Zeiner, H.K., Pollay, M., & Kaplan, R.J. (1983). Neuropsychological functioning in children with shunted uncomplicated hydrocephalus. *Child's Brain, 10,* 112–120.

Radke, J., & Gosky, G.A. (1981). Hearing and speech screening in a hydrocephalus myelodysplasia population. *Spina Bifida Therapy, 3,* 25.

Rahlson, P. (1983). Hyperverbal behavior in children with shunted hydrocephalus and myelomeningocele (Doctoral dissertation, University of Iowa, 1983). *Dissertation Abstracts International, 44* (8-A), 2420–2421.

Rickard, K., Brady, M.S., & Gresham, E.L. (1977). Nutritional management of the chronically ill child: Congenital heart disease and myelomeningocele. *Pediatric Clinics of North America, 24,* 157–174.

Riggins, R.S., Kraus, J., & Fontanetta, P. (1983). Hip dislocations in myelodysplasia: A functional assessment. *Southern Medical Journal, 76,* 736–739.

Riggs, E. (1982). Urinary diversion in the child with meningomyelocele. *Clinical Proceedings: Children's Hospital National Medical Center, 38,* 168–169.

Robinson, J., & Robinson, C. (1978). Sensorimotor functions and cognitive development. In M.E. Snell (Ed.), *Systematic instruction of the moderately and severely handicapped.* Columbus, OH: Charles E. Merrill.

Sand, P.L. Taylor, N., Hill, M., Kosky, N., & Rawlings, M. (1974). Hand function in children with myelomeningocele. *American Journal of Occupational Therapy, 28,* 87–90.

Scherzer, A.L., & Tscharnuter, I. (1982). *Early diagnosis and therapy in cerebral palsy.* New York: Marcel Dekker.

Seligman, M. (1985). Handicapped children and their families. *Journal of Counseling and Development, 64,* 274–277.

Sharrard, W.J. (1983). Management of paralytic subluxation and dislocation of the hip in myelomeningocele. *Developmental Medicine and Child Neurology, 25,* 374–376.

Shepherd, K., Hickstein, R., & Shepherd, R. (1983). Neurogenic faecal incontinence in children with spina bifida: Rectosphincteric responses and evaluation of a physiological rationale for management, including biofeedback conditioning. *Australian Pediatric Journal, 19,* 97–99.

Sheridan, M.D. (1973). *Manual for the STYCAR vision tests.* Berks, England: NFER Publishing.

Shurtleff, D.B. (1983). Various types of surgery may be needed. *Spina Bifida Insights, 11,* 3.

Shurtleff, D.B., Flotz, E.L., & Loeser, J.D. (1973). Hydrocephalus: A definition of its progression and relationship to intellectual function, diagnosis and complications. *American Journal of Diseases of Children, 125,* 688.

Smith, A.J., & Cote, K.S. (1982). *Look at me.* Philadelphia: Pennsylvania College of Optometry Press.

Smithells, R.W., Sheppard, S., Schorah, C.J., Seller, M.J., Nevin, N.C., Harris, R., Read, A.P., & Fielding, D.W. (1980). Possible prevention of neural-tube defects by periconceptual vitamin supplementation. *Lancet, 1,* 339–340.

Soare, P.L., & Raimondi, A.J. (1977). Intellectual and perceptual-motor characteristics of treated myelomeningocele children. *American Journal of Diseases of Children, 131,* 199–204.

Spain, B. (1974). Verbal and performance ability in preschool children with spina bifida. *Developmental Medicine and Child Neurology, 16,* 773–780.

Stephens, S.C. (1983). Disabilities of written language performance among children with spina bifida (Doctoral dissertation, Texas Woman's University, 1983). *Dissertation Abstracts International, 45* (1-B), 121.

Strassburg, M.A., Greenland, S., Portigal, L.D., & Sever, L.E. (1983). A population-based case-control study of anencephalus and spina bifida in a low-risk area. *Developmental Medicine and Child Neurology, 25,* 632–641.

Swinyard, C.A. (1980). *The child with spina bifida.* Chicago: Spina Bifida Association of America.

Swisher, L.P., & Pinsker, E.J. (1971). The language characteristics of hyperverbal hydrocephalic children. *Developmental Medicine and Child Neurology, 13,* 746–755.

Tew, B. (1979). The "cocktail party" syndrome in children with hydrocephalus and spina bifida. *British Journal of Disorders of Communication, 14*, 89–101.

Tew, B.J., & Laurence, K.M. (1975). The effects of hydrocephalus on intelligence, visual perception and school attainment. *Developmental Medicine and Child Neurology, 17*, 129–133.

Tew, B.J., Payne, H., & Laurence, K.M. (1974). Must a family with a handicapped child be a handicapped family? *Developmental Medicine and Child Neurology, 16* (Supplement 32), 95–98.

Turnbull, A., Summers, J., & Brotherson, M. (1983). *Working with families with disabled members: A family systems approach.* Lawrence: University of Kansas.

Uzgiris, I.C., & Hunt, J. McV. (1975). *Assessment in infancy: Ordinal scales of psychological development.* Urbana: University of Illinois Press.

Vernon, M. (1979). Parental reactions to birth-defective children. *Postgraduate Medicine, 65*, 183–189.

Warwick, R., & Williams, P.L. (1973). *Gray's anatomy* (35th ed.). Edinburgh, Scotland: Churchill Livingstone.

Weikart, D. (1971). *The cognitively oriented curriculum: A framework for preschool teachers.* Washington, DC: National Association for the Education of Young Children.

Westby, C.E. (1980). Assessment of cognitive and language abilities through play. *Language, Speech, and Hearing Services in Schools, 11*, 154–168.

Williams, S.R. (1981). *Nutrition and diet therapy* (4th ed.). St. Louis: C.V. Mosby.

Williamson, G.G. (1981). Pediatric overview. In B.C. Abreu (Ed.), *Physical disabilities manual.* New York: Raven Press.

Windham, G.C., & Edmonds, L.D. (1982). Current trends in the incidence of neural tube defects. *Pediatrics, 70*, 333–337.

Wolraich, M. (1983). *The needs of children with spina bifida: A comprehensive view.* Iowa City: University of Iowa.

Yeargan, D.J.R. (1982). A factor-analytic study of adaptive behavior and intellectual functioning in learning disabled children (Doctoral dissertation, North Texas State University, 1982). *Dissertation Abstracts International, 43* (8-A), 2614.

Zeitlin, S. (1981a). Coping, stress, and learning. *Journal of the Division for Early Childhood, 2*, 102–108.

Zeitlin, S. (1981b). Learning through coping: An effective preschool program. *Journal of the Division for Early Childhood, 4*, 53–61.

Zeitlin, S. (1985). *The coping inventory.* Bensenville, IL: Scholastic Testing Service.

Zeitlin, S., Williamson, G.G., & Szczepanski, M. (1986). *Early Coping Inventory.* Edison, NJ: John F. Kennedy Medical Center, Pediatric Rehabilitation Department.

Index

Abdominal muscles
  assessment of control and therapy
    for, 59
  activities to strengthen, 88
Acuity, visual, 121
AFP, *see* Alpha-fetoprotein
Agnosia, 25
Alpha-fetoprotein (AFP), 4–5
Ambulation
  activities to promote, 79
  crutches and, 119
  difficulties due to age, 113
  dislocated hip and, 93
  effect of hip dislocation surgery on,
    91
  parapodium and, 114–115
  predicting child's status in, 113
  training for, 69–78
  see also Mobility
Amniocentesis, 5
Amniogram, 5
Ankle and foot deformities
  described, 95–97
  surgery for, 95
  therapeutic intervention for, 95, 97
Anticholinergic drugs, bladder manage-
    ment and, 173
Apraxia, 27–28
Arnold-Chiari malformation, 4, 21, 29
Assessment
  of child's coping skills, 190–191
  of child's vision, 121–123
  importance of, 18
  sensorimotor
    movement skills and, 38–40

  muscle strength and, 37–38
  muscle tone and, 37
  points to be included in, 35
  postural control and, 40–41
  range of motion and, 35–37
  sensation and, 38
  sensory integrative skills and,
    41–42
  of urinary system, 171–172
  of vestibular processing, 135
  of visual perception, 128–130
  see also Intervention
Astereognosis, 25, 38
Asymmetrical tonic neck reflex, 39–40
Ataxia, cerebellar, 21
Attention span, tactile defensiveness
  and, 25

"Backward chaining" and dressing, 165
Barlows test, 90
Bathing, 168–170
Binocular vision, 20
Bladder, *see* Bowel and bladder
  management
Bowel and bladder management
  assessment of, 171–172
  incontinence and, 3–4
  other problems with, 170–171
  at school, 195–196
  techniques for, 172–174
  see also Urological problems
Braces
  classroom considerations and,
    196–197
  clothing with, 112, 163–168